Emma Jean Tedder, MSW

Understanding and Assisting Low-Income Women with Cancer

Pre-publication
REVIEW

"The most important contribution from this book is that it will heighten the reader's level of sensitivity to the plight of all women who battle cancer.

A new social worker in the field of medical social work, particularly in oncology, will find this to be helpful. It is most suited for the outpatient setting.

As a worker in the acute setting, I found Ms. Tedder's recommendations about posttreatment support groups (i.e., composition, etc.) to be useful and a consideration I will try to integrate into my own work.

I especially appreciated the point about the role of case management and how a multidisciplinary approach is the preferred way of helping an individual throughout the many phases of this illness."

Nancy Strach, LSW
Medical Social Worker,
St. Francis Medical Center,
Honolulu, Hawaii

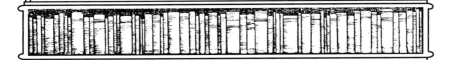

Understanding and Assisting Low-Income Women with Cancer

Understanding and Assisting Low-Income Women with Cancer

Emma Jean Tedder, MSW

The Haworth Press
New York • London

The Haworth Press, Inc., 10 Alice Street, Binghamton, NY 13904-1580

Cover design by Marylouise E. Doyle.

Library of Congress Cataloging-in-Publication Data

Tedder, Emma Jean.
  Understanding and assisting low-income women with cancer / Emma Jean Tedder.
    p.   cm.
  Includes bibliographical references and index.
  ISBN 0-7890-0426-7 (alk. paper).
  1. Cancer in women—Social aspects. 2. Cancer in women—Economic aspects. 3. Poor women—Medical care. 4. Poor women—Diseases. I. Title.
RC281.W65T43 1998
362.1'96994'0082—dc21

                                                                    98-5302
                                                                      CIP

In memory of my best friend
Mary B. Fellion,
who died of cancer,
and her daughter Alice,
who died of cancer at age 17,
and their surviving family,
who have enriched my life.

ABOUT THE AUTHOR

Emma Jean Tedder, MSW, is the Director of Social Work Services at the Charlotte Maxwell Complementary Clinic (CMCC) in Oakland, California, an organization serving low-income women with cancer. She provides support, advocacy, resource development and referral, case management, crisis intervention, and counseling around issues of cancer. She also writes a column for *Charlotte's Web,* the Clinic's newsletter. Besides teaching at CMCC's volunteer trainings, Ms. Tedder provides field instruction to school interns from the School of Social Work at San Francisco State University.

CONTENTS

Foreword

The disease cancer has become well known in our society today. Rare are the individuals whose lives have not been touched by the cancer experience, either their own or that of a family member, friend, or colleague. We know of the disease of cancer—the physical and emotional hardships, the disfigurement, fatigue, and illness that can accompany cancer and its treatments. But although we may think about how an individual copes with cancer and its sequelae, we may not think of the financial cost involved or the physical cost of getting to appointments and treatments. These costs are an added burden that cancer inflicts upon those who have low incomes.

The impact of cancer and its aftermath can be a traumatic experience. But how much more traumatic can it be when one has no family, friends, or an adequate income? Or when your ethnic or cultural background is different from your fellow patients and those who treat you? These are the issues that Jean Tedder focuses on in this book. Drawing on her own experiences as a social worker who has worked extensively with women with cancer, Ms. Tedder discusses the many difficulties of being a low-income woman with cancer. Using the patients' own stories, Ms. Tedder not only illustrates the hardships of facing cancer and its treatment, but also offers examples of how low-income women have dealt with their illness and its aftermath. In addition she offers guidance on how social workers and other therapists may be of help to these women.

I hope that this book will enhance the understanding and respect for the courage with which low-income people face hardships in their lives. In addition, I hope that the suggestions provided by Ms. Tedder are of use to the many people who provide services to those in need.

Ellen G. Levine, PhD, MPH
Clinical (Medical) Psychologist,
Research Director, Psychosocial Oncology,
California Pacific Medical Center,
San Francisco, CA

Acknowledgments

My gratitude and heartfelt thanks to Michael Hawthorne and his magic computer; to my friends who encouraged me; and to everyone who cares about low-income women with cancer.

Smiling in Here?—Elsa and Helen

by Anna

My face smiled from within
on seeing this woman who remembers my name.
I delight in her rebel remarks
and trust her.
She's on my side.

But who's on the other side?
I thought those with scalpels
were cold, heartless,
as metallic as their knives—
incisive precision without mercy.
I thought I would die before letting them carve me.
My life, in MY hands—the lone ranger capable of all.

These women, warm and caring,
have changed me.
I lie down
with their hands on me,
trusting.
My tension gives in, loosens,
as women's hands, under caring eyes,
cut away what my body cannot survive.
Doing for me
what the lone ranger cannot do for herself.

They say yes so often—
"Afraid your ovaries are malignant too?
We'll stay to look at them with you."
As I wilt and cry, she offers herself,
dissolving my despair into caring arms.

1

"Fewer drugs in your body?
How nice that you're informed—
We can do that."

"Maria's hands at your head?
I think we can find a space for her."

Protocol bends here, as they fill a woman's deep need
for touch and self.

My life has changed.
I hope to care for others as these women have cared for me.

I know how it feels to need and be namelessly alone.
When they touched me, with arms and eyes caring,
I remembered: there is someone in here to care for.

Did I hear a bird chirping?
Or was it the spirit of these women?

Chapter 1

The Impact

It is difficult to find writings and/or studies that investigate the combination of low-income women and cancer. However, literature is available to substantiate the meaning of each factor within the context of society. That is to say, we can readily learn what it means to be low-income, apart from being a woman who has cancer. On the other hand, some attention has been given to middle-class women with cancer. Although it is not enough, they do have support groups and resource centers, most of which do not reach out to help women in the lower classes. In fact, it is rare to hear of one that does. Unfortunately, low-income women with cancer have been neglected by their middle-class counterparts and researchers alike. They are nonpersons.

The need for considering this population is as important as longevity itself since death rates due to cancer are higher among poor women in the United States, according to Anderson (1986, p. 73).

Although we acknowledge delay in treatment can result in death and Kosa and colleagues (1969, p. 205) tell us "lower class persons are more likely to delay seeking treatment than higher status persons" a more global view implies that these high death rates may be more closely linked with poverty itself, rather than with one type of behavior alone. Delay in treatment may not be universal among poor people. Also, if poor people could only afford treatment, perhaps they would seek it sooner.

A study in Bursa cited poverty as one of the significant factors responsible for esophageal carcinoma in northeastern Turkey (Memik, Gulten, and Nak, 1992). Likewise, very low income, or subsistence income, was recorded as a risk factor for cervical cancer in Ethiopian women (Pelzer et al., 1992). In Texas, black, white, and Hispanic women all gave "cost" as well as "lack of physician referral" as reasons prior to the study for not having mammography (Vernon, 1992).

Besides the lack of financial resources, the social stigma of poverty has bearing on whether a poor woman survives cancer. As Belle (1982, p. 96) tells us: "Stigmatization makes the individual seem less than human, allows others to explain her difficulties as a result of her inferiority and to exercise discrimination in ways that effectively reduce her life chances." Since discrimination is linked to stigmatization, why focus primarily on poor women—why not poor women and men together?

"Historically, women have suffered from oppression and discrimination simply because of their sex" (Belle, 1982, p. 109). Otherwise—when it is easy to name many emotionally healthy women who have breast cancer—how can the travesty against them be accepted, according to Bacon's (1952/1979) study of forty women which determined the following personality predispositions:

1. A masochistic character structure
2. Inhibited sexually
3. Inhibited motherhood
4. Inability to discharge or deal with anger, aggressiveness, or hostility, covered by a facade of pleasantness
5. An unresolved conflict with the mother, handled through denial and sacrifice
6. Delay in securing treatment (pp. 453-460)

In addition to further stigmatizing women who have cancer, Bacon and her colleagues totally ignore the oppression of women in a society in which rich white men are in power, nor do they consider servitude as a personality predisposition for women in a patriarchal society. Moreover, a sample of forty cannot represent the thousands of women who die every year in this country from cancer, many of whom are poor. Who will speak for them?

In reality, women, particularly poor women with cancer, have shown enormous strength and resourcefulness. They are expected to deal with far more than a male-dominated society might be willing to admit. Furthermore, these women's lives speak for themselves. They have had to do more with less money, make wiser decisions with less education, carry more responsibility with less power, and somehow survive in a society that seems to always find new ways to abuse poor people and which shows little respect for women.

In a medical setting:

> the age group that seemed most difficult for the nursing staff, from the points of view of social loss, family stress, loss of body image, functioning and independence, as well as pain, suffering, and anger were those in their late thirties to early fifties . . . As one patient stated: "I've just got to get home; I have so many responsibilities. My daughters are only fourteen and sixteen; I have a seventeen-year-old son and two older ones. My mother is semi-senile in a nursing home . . ." (Germain, 1979, p. 184)

Further, Anderson (1986, p. 197) tells us women must act as patients and then "leave their cancer in the hospital," which is especially difficult when dealing with the side effects of chemotherapy. They must assume their roles as wives, mothers, workers, and friends. Many have to carry on conflicting roles in a hardship-as-usual life, while they go through an ongoing, overwhelming, multitragic, catastrophic illness that could very well end their lives altogether.

Poor women must do all this—without money, respect, and sometimes without the support of a loving family, which can:

lead the patient to feel rejected or abandoned by loved ones. The patient may also respond to this ambiguous or negative feedback with a lowered sense of self-esteem . . . In some cases cancer patients are "victimized" . . . relationships have become problematic because, rather than providing support for the patient, those around her have isolated, rejected, or even blamed her for the cancer . . . often seen as unclean and sinful in origin . . . (Anderson, 1986, p. 235)

Thence, we are just beginning to understand the impact poverty and its interwoven psychosocial stressors can have on women who are trying to deal with cancer. Cooper (1984, p. 73) says "to employ an engineering term, external stress [persisting situations such as poverty and lack of emotional support] leads to strain on the structure." It is no surprise to find depression, low self-esteem, and financial difficulties among the major problems faced by cancer patients (Stoll, 1979, p. 136). Undoubtedly, these problems become much more intense among those women beset by both cancer and poverty.

Therefore, it is crucial that we ask not only what is the link between all these stressors and cancer, but also what is the most important factor leading to survival and a sense of well-being? Gawler (1987, p. 141) agrees with Cooper (1984), who states:

The animal and human studies of stress, psychoneuro-immunology, and cancer find that effective coping has a striking impact on both tumor development and on immune system-related hormonal changes which can be expected to influence tumor growth. . . . Herein is the potential link between depression and stress in relationship to cancer; studies in both areas are likely to be measuring an inefficient coping style when they report a significant relationship to cancer. . . . In addition, there is clear application of the measure of self-derogation to coping style . . . which seems to reflect a special vulnerability to life stressors. (pp. 44-45)

It does not seem likely that a patriarchal society that disrespects and abuses low-income people, particularly women, through a multitude of financial and social stressors would then provide them with the means to cope. And, it seems even more unlikely that poor women, who rarely name their oppressors, would be able to develop optimal coping styles without help. It is this problem we as social workers must address for women who, stigmatized and deprived by poverty, are struggling against malignant cancer. Beyond that, we need to increase sensitivity toward women of color with cancer because they have an even greater struggle against oppression (Belle, 1982, pp. 109-110).

Fortunately, the number of middle-class women campaigning against cancer is on the rise, as evidenced by the march in Sacramento on Mother's Day 1991. The movement has begun; more efforts will follow. Activism itself is a means of coping.

However, the woman of lower socioeconomic status may not feel comfortable or welcome with the middle-class. She may even feel like an outcast. And when she discovers she has cancer and realizes her life may be cut short, where will she turn? Who will help her cope? Who will speak for her?

Chapter 2

The Aftermath

> Throughout their life, cancer survivors continue to have special medical concerns, preoccupation with fears of recurrence, a sense of greater vulnerability to illness, a pervasive awareness of their own mortality, a more negative view of the future, and a permanent sense of being physically inferior. All remain permanently and conspire to diminish self-assurance and confidence. Concern about infertility often submerged at the time of diagnosis and treatment, reemerges with great power when patients marry, often causing severe distress. (DeVita, Hellman, and Rosenberg, 1989, p. 2202)

Assuming the above observation is correct, why can't cancer survivors simply make the transition from illness to wellness? How can so many people from diverse backgrounds, having been declared well, or cured, or in remission, be different in so many ways from the way they were prior to diagnosis? Having become tumor free, does it matter what the illness was as far as resuming a normal life is concerned? And what about expectations in a society where the strength of the individual is stressed? Are survivors not victorious over their disease? Are some actually lagging behind physically, economically, emotionally, and socially? If so, what do these questions mean to those who work with low-income women in treatment for cancer when that treatment ends?

If we consider the possibility of an aftermath of cancer, we can develop a much better understanding of the low-income female survivor through examining the physical, economic, social, and emotional changes that may have taken place. Although every person may not experience a significant aftermath, there are far more who do than is realized, and economic vulnerability tends to predispose the low-income woman for posttreatment difficulties, regardless of expectations.

To begin, there is an expectation of a simple, prompt transition from illness to wellness that is projected by the medical community and consequently is accepted by family, friends, and society at large. This in itself can be demoralizing to the woman who is experiencing difficulties beyond treatment and who needs to have that experience validated, rather than denied. It is as if there is a cutoff point at the end of treatment that has an expectation of full recovery. And, if the patient still complains of feeling sick, she may be seen as lacking gratitude for having survived.

Actually, gratitude is often accompanied by a myriad of problems that can give one a sense that it is not really over. However, when treatment is deemed successful, cancer and its treatment, along with all the ramifications, seem to be perceived as transient phenomena that are without an aftermath. Perhaps this is due, in part, to the medical profession's fear of lawsuits. Certainly, it complicates "reentry problems at the time of return to normal life" (DeVita, Hellman, and Rosenberg, 1989, p. 2201).

Nevertheless, iatrogenic problems can and do occur:

> Ralph W. Moss, author of *The Cancer Industry,* takes a far different view of chemotherapy in his book. He cites the common side effects of chemotherapy treatment as though they were permanent rather than temporary, going so far as to state, "the use of chemotherapy is often accompanied by the destruction of the immune system." (Reyes, 1991, p. 2)

Moreover, "Orthodox methods have one particularly difficult side effect in common: radiation and chemotherapy both damage the body's immune system" (McGinn and Haylock, 1993, p. 26).

Likewise, it is entirely possible for a survivor to have ongoing symptoms of chronic fatigue immune dysfunction syndrome (CFIDS) that include extreme fatigue; chronic, intermittent sore throat; muscle pain; joint pain; and other flulike symptoms (Bell, 1991, pp. 34-35). Unfortunately, these symptoms are likely to be ignored, unrecognized, or passed over by many doctors who seem to see tumor-free status as synonymous with health. Some even demonstrate an attitude of "Don't complain or you will be viewed as a mental case."

Clearly, the debilitation and misery caused by a poorly functioning body has long-term implications that must be considered when working with this population. Otherwise, it is possible for an uninformed worker to slip into a blame-the-victim stance if the low-income survivor fails to measure up to treatment expectations.

Continuing our focus on posttreatment problems, even the *Merck Manual,* a conservative medical book, admits to posttreatment pain syndromes:

> Post-surgical syndromes: Post-thoracotomy, Post-mastectomy, Post-radical neck, Phantom limb and stump pain.
>
> Post-chemotherapy syndromes: Peripheral neuropathy [nerve damage], aseptic necrosis, [increasing changes] of the femoral [thigh] head, steroid pseudo-rheumatism.
>
> Post-radiation therapy syndromes: Fibrosis of brachial or lumbrosacral plexus, Radiation myelopathy [spinal changes], Radiation necrosis [*changes* from cell death] of bone, Radiation-induced second primary tumors. (Berkow, 1987, p. 1342)

Although it is neither feasible nor desirable to explore in depth every aspect of cancer treatment in our discourse of the aftermath, it is useful to specify the possible incidental side effects of several widely used cancer therapy drugs that can have permanent impact on the individual. This will help us to understand, rather than judge, those women who appear to be too slow in their recovery.

For that reason then we will review Adriamycin, cyclophosphamide, Decadron, and tamoxifen, respectively. Decadron, a strong corticosteroidal drug, is frequently used in conjunction with tumor-destroying drugs such as adriamycin and/or cyclophosphamide during aggressive treatment. Many breast cancer patients are given this combination along with a third drug such as 5-fluorouracil. Tamoxifen, which we might think of as an estrogen blocker, is often prescribed for breast cancer when the aggressive treatment ends and the posttreatment period begins. It is usually taken for a period of five years.

According to the *Physicians Desk Reference* (1993):

Adriamycin [also known as Doxorubicin]
> Congestive heart failure and/or cardiomyopathy may be encountered several weeks after discontinuation of Adriamycin therapy. . . . [It] may potentiate the toxicity of other anti-cancer therapies. (pp. 560-561)

Cyclophosphamide [also known as Cytoxin]
> Cyclophosphamide interferes with oogenesis and spermatogenesis. It may cause sterility in both sexes. . . . [Second malignancies have developed in some patients.] (pp. 744-745)

Then there is Decadron, for which "adverse reactions" are listed. They include but are not limited to:

- Fluid and Electrolyte Disturbances, such as congestive heart failure
- Musculoskeletal, such as fractures
- Gastrointestinal, such as peptic ulcer with possible perforation and hemorrhage
- Dermatologic, such as thin, frail skin, increased sweating, and impaired wound healing
- Neurologic, such as increased intracranial pressure and psychic disturbances

- Endocrine, such as development of cushingoid state [upper body fat, round, moon face, and hump at the back base of the neck], and secondary adrenocortical and pituitary unresponsiveness, particularly in times of stress, as in trauma, surgery or illness
- Ophthalmic, such as glaucoma
- Metabolic
- Cardiovascular, such as myocardial rupture
- Other, such as weight gain (*PDR,* pp. 1498-1499)

Finally, there is tamoxifen (also known as Nolvadex) with its daily, year-after-year side effects: "Visual disturbances including corneal changes, cataracts and retinopathy have been reported . . ." (*PDR,* p. 1127). An additional sixteen adverse reactions are listed. They include menstrual disorder, bone pain, nausea, cough, ede-ma, fatigue, ovarian cyst(s), abdominal cramps, and depression (p. 1128). Not all who take tamoxifen experience all the side effects, but some of these side effects are significant and for some women are so severe that they cannot continue with the drug.

"Of these effects the most serious is depression," and "Therapy to combat side effects is unsatisfactory." Love further states, "possible carcinogenic effects of tamoxifen on the liver should urge caution with respect to long-term use in humans" (1989, p. 809). As one anonymous informed breast cancer survivor expressed: "I take tamoxifen to avoid a recurrence, which my doctor said would be absolutely fatal, but in so doing I risk developing a liver cancer that would also shorten my life. In the meantime, I have to live with ongoing fatigue, nausea, bone pain, and hot flashes."

Besides physical problems, cancer survivors frequently have to live with what can be a disabling economic situation. Having somehow dealt with the loss of personal income, if treatment was too debilitating to allow her to continue working, plus having to absorb treatment-connected expenses such as transportation and clothing for a changed body size, the low-income woman may find herself and her family destitute. Experience reveals a surprising number of women who lose all financial assets, even their apartments, when faced with a diagnosis of cancer and no health insurance. The diagnosis alone costs hundreds of dollars, which can easily break a struggling family. In fact, a middle-class woman is "more apt to become poor than well, since the average cancer treatment costs about $30,000" (Brady, 1991b, p. 25).

When she is finally able to work again, the cancer survivor often encounter job discrimination that has existed for years and still exists today—legal or not. Mellette (1989) tells us; "The Legal Aid Society of San Francisco has documented the existence of some job problems" (p. 101), and DeVita and colleagues (1989) concur: "Discrimination in employment and health insurance coverage is frequent" (p. 2201). Furthermore, "Until AIDS, cancer was the most feared disease of the twentieth century and the one most stigmatized" (Kofron, 1993, p. 41).

If and when energy and stamina return, women surviving cancer often undergo significant changes in their lives. According to Hubner (1989), in a study of 200 women, "Many respondents had experienced major changes in their lives after completing active treatment. Thirty percent had changed jobs, 23 percent had changed their living arrangements, and 8 percent experienced major physical or mental disability" (p. 25).

Besides issues of employment, career, and insurance, those who were out of treatment expressed concern about fertility, personal or intimate physical relations, and discussing their illness with friends, colleagues, and family. "Some people, because of their own fears and conflicts, cannot tolerate the reality of cancer in someone close to them" (McGinn and Haylock, 1993, p. 368).

Frequently, friendships are stressed or ended during treatment:

> There are other kinds of scars. The process of renegotiating relationships may be painful. The friends who could not toler-

ate any part of cancer and dropped from view during the woman's treatment may be gone forever. Other people may continue to treat her differently than they once did. If a support "sister" dies, a woman grieves the loss. (McGinn and Haylock, 1993, p. 364)

Replacing friends, and sometimes even family ties, lost during treatment repeatedly raises difficult questions such as:

- How will new friends react when I tell them I had cancer?
- Will people distance themselves from me out of fear?
- Do I have to always show a Pollyanna attitude and keep any troubling feelings I may have to myself?
- How can I explain feeling sick or fatigued so much of the time when I'm in remission?
- Will they think I'm a hypochondriac or that my problems are psychosomatic?
- If I can't lose the weight I gained during treatment, how will I live with the additional stigma of being fat?

For some, a changed body image brings even tougher questions: If I get into a relationship, will my melanoma scars be a turnoff? What does a man think when a woman tells him she only has one breast? What about physical intimacy after a colostomy? In addition, "Cancer treatment can cause long-term sexual dysfunction in survivors" (DeVita, Hellman, and Rosenberg, 1989, p. 2206). There may also be mixed feelings: "Words women use to describe themselves during and after treatment include victim, ugly, weak, stupid, dependent—and strong, survivor, sensitive, magnificent, focused" (McGinn and Haylock, 1993, p. 36).

Even if a survivor manages to maintain sound emotional health and a high level of self-esteem, she may not be prepared to deal with the emotional fallout that can cling tenaciously long after treatment ends.

> From a psychological perspective, there are no disabling symptoms, but levels of both anxiety and depression are significantly elevated and remain so for years. Some patients reexperienced the anxiety and nausea and vomiting of chemotherapy when exposed to tastes and smells of treatment as long as twelve years later. (DeVita, Hellman, and Rosenberg, 1989, p. 2202)

The above remarks touch upon an aspect of the aftermath that experience shows is entirely possible but difficult, if not impossible, to document in a search of the literature. The *symptoms* of full-blown post-traumatic stress disorder (PTSD) resulting from extreme fear of chemotherapy (which may feel like facing death day after day for months) can go undiagnosed for years and subsequently be left untreated, leaving the cancer survivor dangling from her own emotional limb of fear with nothing to cling to, reliving again and again the nightmares of her own mortality. From the point of view of such a person, living through a major earthquake would seem a very minor disturbance indeed (American Psychiatric Association, 1987, pp. 247-251, 384-385).

Another fear, the fear of recurrence, of having to go through it all again, is another part of the aftermath. And when one's doctor declares a recurrence will surely be fatal, it is similar to a death sentence. Therefore, we can understand how experiencing the aftermath of cancer makes the quality of life such an important issue. As Mellette (1989) tells us:

> Cancer survivors want more than just life. Each patient is a candidate for cancer rehabilitation—the process of preventing or ameliorating the physical and psychosocial dysfunctions that result from cancer or its treatment. (p. 93)

Since the efficacy of the support group is common knowledge among social workers and is discussed elsewhere in this writing, there is no need to document that here, nor to delve deeply into the characteristics and standards needed for a successful post-treatment group. Suffice it to say then that probably the most important service we can provide to this population is the post-treatment support group because it can end isolation, reduce stress, and empower the individual to investigate and access other resources as she needs them.

For the low-income woman, the team approach for rehabilitation would be ideal because poverty renders one more vulnerable overall. More important, she who needs the services most is least able to access them or to even know such services might exist at all.

As an example of the team approach, the Cancer Rehabilitation and Continuing Care Program at the Medical College of Virginia has been operative since the 1970s. This program includes a physician, a coordinator trained in rehabilitation counseling, two physical therapists, two occupational therapists, another rehabilitation counselor, a speech pathologist, four home care nurses, and two social workers for home care, a part-time dietitian, a music therapist, plus volunteers and home health aids. It is a matter of continuing care that, as with treatment itself, is tailored to the individual's needs (Mellette, 1989, p. 103).

Ultimately, in the multisided ruins of the aftermath of cancer that is so poorly understood by so many, it behooves us to provide supportive services that not only reclaim lives, but also extend as far beyond the end of treatment as the person needs. And, we must include all survivors, particularly the more vulnerable low-income woman—for there is not one among us who will escape being deeply touched in some way by cancer during our lifetimes.

Chapter 3

Three Interviews

If we are to understand and assist low-income women who have cancer, we need to look beyond the literature to the women themselves. Their needs and concerns as seen by *them* are essential to the healing process as it applies to the development of self-determination and the mind-body connection.

Therefore, three interviews were conducted (separately, but discussed here together), so that we can observe the impact and aftermath of cancer diagnosis and treatment, comparing these women with each other as well as with their middle-class counterparts.

As it turned out, none of the three women interviewed have experienced chemotherapy or radiation. A year ago at age thirty-seven, Lucia, a charming and gracious lesbian woman, was diagnosed with uterine cancer, which was treated surgically with a complete hysterectomy. Diane, an African American, has just celebrated her second year of remission from breast cancer for which she underwent a mastectomy. A caring, single parent of two teenage boys, she is forty years of age. Clare was diagnosed with melanoma sixteen years ago at the age of twenty-four. Her primary illness was followed by metastasis two years later. Her melanoma was treated surgically both times. Clare is a single woman with three siblings. Determined to rise above poverty, she has struggled to work her way through both undergraduate and graduate school.

Although Lucia, Diane, and Clare are diverse in background as well as in site diagnosis, they have all experienced firsthand what it means to be low-income for a period of time in excess of twenty years, *and* their psychosocial responses to cancer are strikingly similar.

Their initial reaction to a cancer diagnosis was one of fear and a sense of the loss of control over their lives, followed by a desire to know more about their illness, which to some extent is similar to what a middle-class woman experiences. Likewise, they saw access to information as important. The impact of the diagnosis differed for them in that it was accompanied by the belief that cancer is usually fatal. This belief was strongest in Diane: "The word [cancer] itself meant death to me. It was just like hearing the word AIDS. Immediately, my thoughts went to death."

Offsetting this is the hope that certain lifestyle changes will help increase their chances of getting well. When asked what kinds of changes, Diane focused on diet and exercise, while Clare suggested spiritual development, using reading materials, meditation, visualization, support groups, nutrition, rapport with one's physician, and belief in treatment. Unlike the majority of low-income women, Clare's suggestions sound similar to what we might expect to hear from middle-class women. First, one has to be aware of options, and then the same access that middle-class women are more accustomed to, needs to be made available to the lower class. On the other hand, Lucia said, "Most (self-help methods) require access to money, information, help from others, and also self-confidence, time and energy, a sense of hope about the future, which is difficult when life is already burdened with low-income, low social status, and few options for success in anything." Thus, we can see how the low-income woman must first deal with economic and social barriers, and sometimes low self-esteem, before she can avail herself of supportive measures.

Clare also expressed problems with access as a single, low-income woman without close family ties: "I mostly needed emotional support, someone to listen to me, and I didn't get that." As we might expect, an absence of support brings on "profound lonely panic" (Lucia). Although Diane lacked access to supportive services in the beginning, she was able to reach out to family: "I felt that my family could not deal with it [cancer], and with my being a caretaker all my life, I felt I just couldn't handle it and they would worry about me. So it was real hard to let them share this, but I was really surprised what happened when I did." Then Lucia shows us how getting support is a means of accepting responsibility for oneself:

Getting practical support was the absolute most important part of my self-healing. After that, getting emotional support by talking with friends and finding a support group of other women with cancer . . . that has been invaluable to me, not only for emotional support, but for informational sharing. Women with cancer share vital information that cannot be found in books or other media, certainly not from doctors.

In "The Impact," we saw how women with cancer are often unable to temporarily relinquish their familial responsibilities in order to focus on self-care. Similarly, Diane worried about taking care of her dependent children, which is even more of a stressor when faced by a low-income, single parent: "I have a responsibility and they were first in my mind. . . . The first thing I thought about: I can't do this. What's going to happen to my family?" Clare also felt a sense of responsibility, but in a different way. Without strong emotional support, she felt she had to take care of others' feelings about her disease in addition to her own, including siblings, friends, and work associates. Lucia, on the other hand, was disabled at the time of her diagnosis. Being already unable to work because of chronic fatigue immune dysfunction syndrome (CFIDS) and multiple chemical sensitivities (MCS), her sense of responsibility was to herself. She also had the support of friends within the lesbian community. Again, this may not be typical, as she points out: "I am lucky. I know of [low-income] lesbians who've dealt with serious illness alone and sometimes [were] homeless as well."

Beyond treatment, there is a need for ongoing support for low-income women, even those who have not undergone chemotherapy and radiation and whose physical recovery time can be expected to be shorter. They have an aftermath experience that is largely due to the emotional and physical changes imposed by the cancer itself and the resulting surgery. Unlike the middle-class, these women have no financial resources to support them in the event of a recurrence, making the threat of metastasis that much worse: "I have that fear that the cancer can come back. . . . How could I handle it? I have these fears. I try not to think about it" (Diane). Lucia lives "with an increased level of fear, an undercurrent that never completely goes away. . . . I don't know how to put into words the profound effects having cancer has had on me—it's an immense encounter with death."

The low-income woman's aftermath includes a combination of poverty and the stigma of having had cancer: "I still feel like there's a stigma and I won't be seen as a person, if they [new acquaintances] know my history, and will be standoffish if I tell them. So I wait a long time before I tell them" (Clare).

When there are no financial resources for counseling, the stigma and surgical scars can have a psychologically crippling effect. And, for those who are alone, the possibility of ever having an intimate relationship again may seem hopeless. Regarding her mastectomy, Diane said, "I feel like I can't be intimate with anyone. . . . When I look at myself, it's not a pretty sight to me, and so I have a real problem adjusting to that." Clare tells us:

> It was really hard for me to start dating again. How was I going to tell the person, and when? . . . I tried getting help about sexuality issues and body image issues. I saw a counselor just once and the program was disbanded. They just cut the funds. . . .
>
> It's like having a big, huge hole in my leg, and with melanoma people can't have plastic surgery. . . . They can't fill in the holes.

Finally, there are the all-important job and insurance issues, which for low-income women literally mean survival, rather than simply maintaining a middle-class lifestyle. Understandably, these issues complicate the problem of when to disclose a history of cancer. Although discrimination in hiring practices is illegal, it is very difficult to prove, particularly when one cannot afford a lawyer. The inability to secure a job or the loss of one due to cancer puts these women at risk for homelessness. In addition to this stressor, health insurance is financially out of reach, unless it can be obtained through an employer who carries a group policy. Individual policies may have a two-year waiting period for coverage of a recurrence when there is a history of cancer. This is totally unacceptable in view of the low-income woman's risks.

Lucia, as a disabled person, found MediCal coverage difficult: "If I hadn't gotten help from my friends, I'd be sunk. I was already just getting by, and now I needed money for the Sharecost on my MediCal to pay for my [frequent] medical checkups." Cancer patients in remission must accommodate frequent medical exams. Clare's aftermath included being stuck in the same low-paying job: "I was so afraid I couldn't pass a physical and get a job somewhere else . . . so I didn't change jobs for ten years." Conversely, survival may entail a complete job change, particularly for a breast cancer/lymphedema patient who can no longer do physically demanding work, which was Diane's experience. Fortunately, her employer permitted her to move to a desk job from a janitorial position. Having already been through so much, it was frightening for her to undergo new training at that particular time. Although she was able to make the change, Diane's lymphedema still presents problems to be dealt with daily for the rest of her life.

At least, in recent years, the Americans with Disabilities Act (ADA) supports the efforts of those trying to rehabilitate themselves after cancer, regardless of class. That is to say, according to the law, employers must make reasonable accommodations for disabled workers. This may mean shorter, more flexible hours, or necessary equipment purchase or modification. And, it is a mistake to assume that thousands of low-income women with a history of cancer are not suffering some kind of disability. Unfortunately, many suffer in silence, which can be a serious problem when we recall that cancer and its treatment can damage the immune systems of women already struggling with the financial and physical hardships of poverty.

Furthermore, as a society, we need to drop the prevailing get-over-it attitude and begin thinking of cancer as a chronic disease that can often have an extensive aftermath as well as its metastatic occurrence.

Although some low-income women are able to walk away after an encounter with this disease, many cannot. Most will need various kinds of support well beyond their initial treatment.

Looking toward recovery, we can see there is an overall consensus between the interviews and the literature reviewed. In "The Impact" we discovered that having or developing effective coping skills (or ego strengths) is a major psychoneuroimmunological key that turns on the body's ability to fight tumor growth. And, throughout the interviews we get a sense of how each woman called upon all her coping skills, and when that was not enough, reached out to acquire more. The point is that although each woman's physical and social situation was different from the other, all three were somehow able to shift their focus from cancer to coping.

In "The Aftermath" the literature presented posttreatment problems such as fear of recurrence, physical iatrogenic difficulties, changes in relationships with others, and economic setbacks related to employment and insurance. Likewise, the women interviewed spoke of fear, physical changes, scars, reluctance toward intimacy, and job changes.

Lucia, Diane, and Clare have provided us with insight into some of the problems encountered by low-income women with cancer that must be dealt with in addition to problems faced by their middle-class counterparts. Besides having financial problems interlaced with health insurance difficulties, they experienced major obstacles in accessing services. Their success in coping was largely the result of having a strong sense of self—that is to say, a sense that one's own self is worth holding onto. There was also enough physical and emotional energy and stamina to struggle against the odds, so to speak. However, these women are not necessarily typical. There are scores of low-income women who have been so beaten down throughout their lives that, when cancer develops, they lack the emotional energy to struggle or to generate what might be seen as the fighting spirit.

One only has to compare the oncology waiting room of a county hospital with that of a university hospital. Not all, but many low-income women treated at a county hospital tend to suffer in silence. They often appear apathetic, even hopeless, as if waiting to die. By contrast, middle-class women being treated for cancer at a university hospital are much more likely to come together in informal support groups while waiting for treatments. Instead of just accepting without question whatever is prescribed to them, they complain about their doctors not giving them enough time for their questions and not showing consideration for their feelings. They study information about their disease, inquire about treatment options, and may avail themselves of supportive alternative therapies. In other words, they do not accept a cancer diagnosis as a death sentence but, rather, are more inclined to rally all their forces and activate well-developed coping skills.

Our goals are clear. If we are to assist low-income women with cancer to overcome an immobilized state of crisis, to stabilize them, and to empower them toward wellness, we must pay attention to self-esteem issues and help them develop positive coping skills, and we must provide access to services. To further bridge the gap between them and the considerations normally reserved for the middle and upper-middle classes, we should first be advised by one who has experienced the journey of cancer as a low-income woman. For this reason, Lucia's suggestions for us who want to help are recorded in her own words, as follows:

- First, ask women directly what they need, and trust that they do know what they need. Then think about other things they might need that they may be used to doing without or might not know about.
- Be very well informed and up to date about all services and funds available, and find ways to get them to women quickly. With cancer, time is always pressing and bureaucracies move much too slowly.
- Women will feel less scared if a social worker makes it clear that she understands what's needed and will do everything in her power to provide it. If something is not available, acknowledge that it should be.
- Be aware that all delays are frightening . . . an hour or a day waiting for services can feel like an eternity. Return phone calls as soon as you can.
- I was upset to find out how hard it was for me to ask for what I needed, even though my life was at stake. . . . I've had a lifetime of being put down, ridiculed, dismissed, and denied necessities. . . . [It's been] very hard to deal with anyone in authority, including social workers. . . . Keep offering help and giving reassurances that women have a right to services.

We will do well to follow Lucia's advice.

Chapter 4

Maria's Case History

At the time of her diagnosis, Maria was about to celebrate her forty-ninth birthday. She had been born into an East Coast, blue-collar family that was dominated by alcoholism, violence, and poverty. Having single-parented a cerebral-palsied child into an independent adulthood, every birthday for her was another step into what she described to her friends as the Part II of her life—the adventure part.

It was with this spirit of adventure that, six months earlier, Maria had moved from San Francisco to North Carolina to take up a new life surrounded by family. She had planned this move many months in advance and had experienced increased longing as she listened to the welcoming voice of her sister during their numerous phone calls. Maria was sure of the emotional support she would need during the adjustment of such a drastic change.

Upon arriving and establishing herself in the community, Maria quickly found a network of business and professional women who were eager to give her job leads and also to welcome her into their social lives.

By contrast, Maria found her family was far more dysfunctional than she had remembered, or perhaps had wanted to remember. As in her childhood, only more so, she was assigned the role of an inferior—a role that was now incongruent with the personal growth she had worked so hard on, both in and out of therapy, during her twelve years in California. She had changed, but her family hadn't.

It was in the midst of a constant barrage of put-downs from her sister and her sister's husband that Maria discovered a lump in her breast during a routine self-examination. She was astonished to find it. Remembering she still had a few months health insurance with an HMO carrying over from her civil service job in California, she immediately asked her sister to help her get to the nearest facility, which was about seventy miles away. The response to her request was described later by Maria as "a drop-dead look."

Maria felt too stressed to deal with yet another problem. She was driving for the first time in twelve years in an unfamiliar place and frequently got lost. She was looking for an apartment so she could remove herself from the oppressive atmosphere of her sister's home as quickly as possible. And, she was working one full-time job, plus a part-time job for survival while she looked for a third job that would use her hard-earned degree and would also offer health insurance. Maria was expending a lot of energy in her job search—energy she felt she didn't have.

She didn't feel well. As a result of these stressors and remembering that benign cysts occurred with some frequency in her family, Maria decided to wait. She was already lining up a position managing a countywide transit system for elderly and disabled people that carried health insurance.

While waiting for a starting date on this new job, Maria quit her other jobs and flew back to San Francisco for a visit, reasoning that it would be a full year before she could take a vacation.

Once there, she was able to think more clearly and to come to terms with the fact that her familial problems would not soon be resolved, if ever. Six months passed and she became more mired in these problems and as a result she became extremely angry. She felt she could not negotiate with closed minds and, worst of all, cold hearts. At that point she returned, packed her belongings, said good-bye to her mother, and moved back to San Francisco.

Maria later said the one benefit of those hellish six months was the friendship she had been able to establish with her mother for the first time in her life.

Having lined up yet another job in San Francisco, Maria used the last of her savings to visit a breast clinic. The lump she had been afraid to touch, since she first discovered it, had doubled in size to an 8 x 8 centimeter tumor. A week later, the clinic called to tell Maria she had breast cancer, Stage III, possibly Stage IV.

Maria was staying with her adult son until she could get reestablished. However, when she told her new employer of the results of the needle aspiration, she was immediately released from that job and so had no income. It was apparent that she would have to stay with her son longer than first expected, much to his dismay over his sense of invaded privacy. It was a studio apartment, and Maria slept on the floor in the kitchen area for the first couple of months, until her son offered to trade places so Maria could have the only bed.

Thus she began treatment at a county hospital, having been referred there after telling the nurse practitioner at the breast clinic that she (Maria) had no income. After her first round of chemotherapy—Adriamycin, Cytoxan, and 5-FU—Maria realized she would be unable to work during treatment.

Feeling weak and fearful, Maria was caught in a downpour of rain while searching for the Department of Social Services. Too weak to stand in line as required, she was able to get the attention of a worker who arranged for a home visit so Maria could apply for General Assistance, which loaned her an income of $285 a month. She then applied for MediCal, a long, arduous task, followed by the first visit to a Social Security office to apply for Supplemental Security Income (SSI). She felt the Social Security representative treated her as a criminal and was fearful her application would be delayed as a result of the worker's attitude, so Maria wrote to Senator Cranston requesting processing assistance. Four months later her SSI benefits materialized. To describe Maria as exhausted throughout her ordeal would be an understatement.

As with many low-income women diagnosed with cancer, after suffering layer upon layer of extraordinary stresses, Maria was plunged into depression. She found herself frequently crying in public with or without provocation. At home, when her son tried to discuss a problem with her, she shrieked that she couldn't deal with his problems and that she didn't want to be his mother anymore. Nights were mostly sleepless. The tumor had become painful, and Maria couldn't stop thinking about her insidious disease that she thought was sure to result in death. When her oncologist told her she had a 15 percent chance of being alive in five years, but not necessarily tumor free, Maria began to wonder just how much time she actually did have.

Her depression deepened; her fear increased. It seemed no one would be able to understand her grief, nor could she control it. Too weak to look for a support group or to drag herself to it if she had found one, Maria was forced to struggle to provide herself with basics as best she could. It took what seemed a superhuman effort to get to her numerous medical appointments, buy groceries and carry them home, do housework, launder her clothes, and keep track of which pills to take and when, around the clock—which is no small feat when there are seven or eight medications.

Treatment was physically and emotionally devastating. On her trips to chemotherapy, she was too weak to stand waiting for a bus and had to find a place to sit. Afraid she might collapse on the street, she worried about having the strength to make it to the hospital. Once there, treatment was at least tedious and frequently painful. Her veins were small; they kept collapsing. It often took forty-five minutes or an hour to insert an IV needle. One nurse after another would try. Sometimes the needle would have to be inserted into Maria's great toe. A small needle had to be used, so another couple hours went by while the liquid slowly dripped.

Fear became a major problem. As soon as she entered the elevator following a treatment, she felt the fear welling up inside of her. Her thoughts reflected this fear: Will I die on the elevator? Will I die while I wait for the taxi? In the cab she would dread the thought of dying there. At home she felt like she was drowning in fear because she was alone.

Maria was not prepared to lose friends at a time when she most needed them. Several removed themselves from Maria's life after hearing of her diagnosis. She felt they were avoiding her and so did not try to hold onto them. A few others dropped her when she became too weak to participate in social activities. One friend talked publicly about Maria's cancer, causing her unnecessary discomfort and embarrassment. Maria broke off the friendship after stating her reasons for doing so. That left two close friends who lived in the area, plus some lifetime friends in various other states, her parents, and her brother.

Those who remained in her life were a great comfort to Maria, because they showed concern. Although Maria established new friendships both during and after treatment, they were mostly women with cancer. Not many of these friends lived, and Maria was often left as mourner. Maria found it difficult to find other friends. She felt people pulled away from her when they learned of her cancer, but it was such a major part of her life, she didn't really know how to avoid disclosure. One could say that cancer actually was her life for quite a long time, and the experience was isolating.

About four months into treatment, Maria was able to acquire an apartment in Senior HUD housing. Being totally alone, her fear increased. Home alone after chemotherapy, with her apartment door closed behind her, she would be afraid to sleep. She thought if she did, she might forget to wake in time to take her meds or, worse, she might die there alone. Every time she awoke she thought: "I'm still alive. Will I live through the day?" Eventually, the nurses at the hospital took turns calling Maria once each day for two days following treatments to see if she was all right. This gave her tremendous relief and also the feeling that she could live between calls. The chemotherapy was more fearful to her than the cancer. Having read that more people die from it, she saw its threat as more immediate.

Throughout her nine months of treatment, Maria was given supportive drugs. As she recalls, they included Elavil for depression, Ativan, Benadryl, Reglan, quarts of Maalox, and Decadron, a strong steroid, plus others she doesn't recall. She was also treated intermittently for chemo-induced thrush and infections resulting from low white cell count. Her immune system was damaged temporarily at least and perhaps for the long term.

She experienced dry mouth and a thirty-pound weight gain from the Elavil. This was in addition to the forty pounds she had gained living with emotional stress caused by her sister and family. Although weight gain had long been a problem for Maria, she had heretofore managed a fair amount of control. However, as treatment continued, Maria found the only thing that felt good in her stomach was peppermint patties, and she acquired another twenty pounds of weight. Discomfort was constant and worsened as the side effects from chemotherapy proved to be cumulative. Convulsively violent retching came in waves within hours of the first injection. Otherwise, when Maria sat, she felt nauseous. When she tried to sleep, she had heartburn. And when she stood, she felt that her legs might buckle beneath her.

She developed an exaggerated dowager's hump and a round, moonlike face from the Decadron. Later, she was to experience skin discoloration from the 5-FU and photosensitivity. Her hair fell out by the handfuls. She tried desperately to attach enough of it on tape so she could wear a scarf and look as if she had bangs showing from beneath it, but failed. She had to buy a wig. To keep her spirits up, she joked about sitting around waiting for her hair to fall out, but inside she was traumatized. It gave her a full, unavoidable realization of how very ill she really was. Looking in the mirror, she felt she saw an ugly stranger.

Shortly after diagnosis, Maria had called her former therapist and made the first of many weekly appointments. She knew she needed all the support she could find. Later she was referred to another therapist who had had cancer and who could teach her visualization. Maria had already tried visualizing her oncologist on her left and her soon-to-be surgeon on her right literally fighting off cancer cells with baseball bats. This became exhausting. Maria needed a technique that wouldn't continue to drain her seriously depleted physical and emotional resources. So in just one session, the therapist guided her into letting her mind produce a picture of the cancer cells sitting in an opposite chair. To Maria they looked like pink sponges.

She spoke to them, first in fear, then in anger. They weakened, dissolving into nothing. She knew then that she could aggressively attack the cancer, and she began to think of herself as a warrior, "a tough old warrior bird." This was Maria's turning point.

Maria's oncologist had explained that the plan was to shrink the tumor to an operable size with chemotherapy, perform a mastectomy, and follow through with six weeks of radiation. Each round of chemotherapy shrunk the tumor two centimeters, far more than had been anticipated. After the third round, Maria was placed on the schedule for surgery. One week before the appointed date, she went to the hospital and was examined thoroughly by several doctors, none of whom could find any sign of the tumor. It was gone, and the doctors were at a loss for an explanation.

For the first time since diagnosis, Maria felt encouraged to hope for continued life. She began to talk of being among the 15 percent who would be alive at the end of five years as described by her doctor earlier—15 percent, that is, of women in Maria's exact medical situation, understanding that every case is different.

The side effects of chemotherapy, however, continued to accumulate, and Maria felt increasingly sicker. Dragging herself to her therapist after the third round, Maria sat and cried during the entire session. She was unable to articulate her feelings, except for saying she could not go on. She could no longer force herself to take the chemotherapy, even though she knew that it was the only insurance available against a fatal recurrence. She was too terrified, too exhausted, and too debilitated. Never in her life had she felt so ill for so long a time. So, although Maria had reached a turning point in her treatment and for the first time since its inception saw hope on the horizon, she felt she could not continue. One might say she experienced the high point just as she hit bottom.

Fortunately, Maria's therapist suggested hypnotherapy to help Maria through the remaining rounds of treatment. Gathering herself together at the end of the session, Maria went home and began looking for a hypnotherapist in the phone book. After many calls in which she repeatedly explained her physical, emotional, and financial situation, Maria found a hypnotherapist at a nearby hospital who, working on her doctorate, needed work with a client in chemotherapy to include in her dissertation. She agreed to see Maria at no charge, and their weekly sessions began.

There were some difficulties such as the long, steep staircase Maria had to climb to the office, wondering each time if her legs could do it and then somehow making it to the top. The hypnotherapy itself helped, but by no means could it be regarded as a panacea. Maria was able to get to her chemotherapy treatments at the hospital. Although she had originally felt safe there, her increased fear began to invade that space as well as at home. At times her fear was replaced by an emotional numbness, and she vacillated between the two feelings. During the treatments, she listened to tapes the hypnotherapist had prepared for her and was able to relax her otherwise taut muscles to some extent. However, as soon as she stepped into the elevator, her mind reverted back to the full-blown thoughts of death described earlier. The fear was always waiting for her, torturing her by day and invading her nights with dreams of mutilated, dismembered bodies.

When Maria's tumor disappeared, a meeting was arranged for Maria, her oncologist, and the surgeon to discuss a mastectomy, which the surgeon still recommended. The oncologist seemed neutral about the decision, leaving it up to Maria. It was explained that if there was a recurrence in that same breast, it would require a major operation involving the sewing in of a large skin flap. There was a 30 percent chance of this happening. Maria, who felt those odds were in her favor, asked if an immediate mastectomy would lengthen her life. The surgeon said "No," and Maria decided right then not to have it. Her treatment plan was adjusted to begin six weeks of radiation while continuing with chemotherapy, with the exception of Adriamycin, which would be added back in after radiation.

Maria's radiation was administered at a university hospital where five days a week she found herself in the ladies waiting room surrounded by women, many of whom were from outside San Francisco. All had cancer; all were frightened. Together they formed an informal support group. For the first time, Maria did not feel alone. It was also her first opportunity to compare her treatment with others'. She was dismayed to find that the tender, loving care given at her clinic in a county hospital was not the norm in other middle-class facilities. On the contrary, it was rare. Most of the women she met spoke of a need for information that was not forthcoming from their male doctors, who had very little time for them and showed even less concern. At best, the women found them patronizing.

About ten months after her diagnosis, Maria went to the clinic for her tenth and last round of chemotherapy. By then her veins were in poor condition. The nurses worked for two and a half hours trying to find a vein that could be used for an IV. They were unsuccessful. The alternative would involve surgery to install a port in her chest. Maria's doctor came in and gave Maria a choice between the surgery and skipping that last round. Maria immediately got out of the bed and gratefully said, "I'm out of here!" It was the end of treatment, but not the end of Maria's story. She had yet to deal with the aftermath.

Having finished chemotherapy, Maria expected to also be finished with fear. The following months proved her wrong. She soon realized the fear remained. She kept experiencing an intermittent feeling of emotional numbness. Sometimes she felt as if she wasn't in her body at all but was simply observing herself, as a functioning but nonfeeling individual. Then, whenever she visited the clinic for her frequent checkups, rode the bus that she had ridden during treatment, or saw the sunlight coming in the bathroom window a certain way, she felt the fear lodged in the pit of her stomach alternating with that out-of-body feeling. There were any number of little reminders that brought the fear back when she least expected. She spoke of this only to her therapist, worrying that others might think her mentally unbalanced.

After treatment, Maria also expected her strength and energy to return. Her doctor expected recovery within a month, but it didn't happen. Maria was still so exhausted that she had to spend most of three or four days a week in bed. And she still did not have the strength to wait for a bus without finding a place to sit.

In addition, she began having severe side effects from the tamoxifen she was now told she would have to take for the rest of her life. Besides being drenched with sweat fifteen to twenty times daily, she was stricken with paralyzingly painful muscle cramps, occurring one after the other. She said if there had been a fire during one of these, she could never have escaped because they were so severe.

Maria's doctor prescribed a number of drugs consecutively to remedy the situation, but the side effects of those were intolerable. At one point, Maria began experiencing neurological symptoms including numbness in her feet. Drifting to the right as she walked, she would sometimes brush against hallway walls. Frequently, when she had to change buses, she became confused and unable to recall where she was going or the next bus to take to get there, even though she had traveled these routes for years.

Suspecting new tumors, Maria's doctor ordered a series of tests. All were negative. She was then referred to a neurosurgeon who diagnosed polyneuropathy, a progressive nerve disorder. He thought it was chemotherapy induced. Finally, in desperation, Maria threw out her meds, except for the tamoxifen, and began taking aspirin daily before the muscle cramps started. It worked. The cramps were fewer as well as much less severe, and the neurological symptoms disappeared except for one that had started during the last two months of treatment. Maria's limbs jerked involuntarily, often, and unexpectedly. Her doctor could not explain it. After about a year, it occurred less frequently and eventually stopped. Maria thinks it was her body's way of responding to fear because she could never relax.

Maria became discouraged over her debilitating fatigue. Whenever she tried to overcome it, she developed sore throat with tender glands and body ache that became severe unless she immediately went to bed for two or three days. When her doctor could find nothing wrong and suggested Maria lose weight, Maria felt ashamed. Thinking she must be a hypochondriac, Maria worked hard at dieting and exercise, but she got worse. She contracted pneumonia, was treated, recovered from that, but did not improve otherwise. She felt she was at fault and if she could only lose weight she would feel well.

Unable to get through the day without large amounts of chocolate for energy, Maria could not manage her weight. The fatigue was so extreme. Finally, she went to a university hospital to see a psychiatrist and tried to describe her fatigue and the fear that would not go away. He referred her to an inexperienced doctor for an evaluation. Several sessions later, Maria was told she was depressed but not seriously enough to be treated there at that clinic. She was advised to continue therapy to work on the related issues and she was then referred to a psychiatrist in private practice, the only one known to accept MediCal. He prescribed Prozac, saying Maria's fatigue was caused by major depression. When she did not improve, he raised the dosage twice. To this, he added lithium at a low dosage.

Maria continued therapy, complaining that her mild, not major, depression came from fatigue and not the reverse. She said that all she needed to be happy was enough energy to carry on her life, and that on days when her energy was better, she felt fine emotionally, even hopeful. Then her energy would fall, and she was back to an intermittently chronic sore throat and body pain.

Eventually, after much sorting, discussion, and some reading, Maria and her therapist agreed that Maria actually had post-traumatic stress disorder (PTSD) along with chronic fatigue immune system dysfunction syndrome (CFIDS), both resulting from her struggle with cancer. They further discovered that depression is part of the constellation of CFIDS symptoms. Maria was greatly relieved to have her feelings validated and to have an experienced professional, who was well-versed in emotional disorders, see her as a normal person. However, when the therapist presented these findings to Maria's oncologist, the doctor stated she did not believe in CFIDS. In fact, it was years before Maria could find a medical doctor who diagnosed and treated the CFIDS.

The psychiatrist who had been prescribing Maria's meds discontinued his practice. Instead of replacing him, Maria gradually reduced the lithium and Prozac until they were eliminated entirely. She began resting more when she was tired and started taking vitamin supplements.

Five years have passed since Maria's diagnosis of breast cancer. Still in remission, she continues regular checkups with her new oncologist, since her original one had relocated. The fatigue, though improved, continues. Much of the weight remains, and the PTSD still haunts her on occasion. Unfortunately, the stigma resulting from the misdiagnosis of major depression shadows Maria via medical records. Maria left psychotherapy, stating she couldn't think of anything more to work on except physical wellness. Prior to leaving, there was a discussion about what she would like to do with the rest of her life. She returned to school on a part-time basis to earn an MSW and now works with low-income women who have cancer.

Maria is deeply grateful to both of the oncologists who literally saved her life. She does hope, however, that a reliable test for CFIDS diagnosis will soon be developed—one that every doctor can believe.

Chapter 5

Maria's Interview on Psychotherapy

Considering the interrelationship of poverty, stress, cancer, effective coping, and psychoneuroimmunology, it behooves us to examine Maria's psychotherapy experience.

As it happens, Maria's sense of self, which in turn gave her the ability to become proactive, came about through psychotherapy. Chronologically, the basis for her healing actually preceded her cancer. That is to say, if Maria's tumor had developed before her search for self in therapy, she would have been one of the majority of low-income women with cancer discussed earlier, who appear to be hopelessly waiting for death to do its work.

Maria describes for us a painful frame of mind when she entered therapy:

> At the beginning, I thought I was less than nothing . . . really low in self-esteem. . . . I didn't have a whole lot of control over my life. It seemed I was pretty much a victim of life. . . . I spent a lot of energy trying to cope with people putting me down. . . . Whenever I tried to make my life better, it never seemed to work out. . . . I felt beaten down.

Rather than falling short by concluding that psychotherapy is the answer to assisting low-income women with cancer, we will be better equipped if we examine the dynamics within the helping relationship and if we understand that these same conditions can be successfully applied not just *in* psychotherapy, but outside as well.

According to Maria, there were five things her therapist did that acted as a catalyst to Maria's transformation. They are at once so simple as to be overlooked, yet so profound as to be life changing. They are: listening, validation, support, space to make one's own decisions, and most important, acceptance.

> I knew I wouldn't be judged. She talked instead about how I could take care of myself. . . . I had never heard of taking care of me. . . . And I always felt like she considered me as an individual and as a worthy person.
>
> It was okay for me to feel whatever came up and to think things through and make my own decision, even if that was different from what others thought I should do.
>
> She always said "What about you? What do *you* want?" That was a new concept to me—thinking that I'm supposed to get something out of life. . . .
>
> I always knew she was on my side, and from that I was able to develop tools for living and strategies to solve problems. . . . I learned to set limits with people.

Thus we can see that Maria's metamorphosis from feeling like "less than nothing" to a strong sense of self is what not only allowed her self-trust, but empowered her to the extent that she could even deal with a catastrophic illness, knowing that her life was worth living.

Moreover, this acquired sense of self is what likens Maria to Clare, Diane, and Lucia. And, although all four women have been low-income throughout most of their lives, they were as proactive in dealing with the impact of cancer as their middle-class counterparts. Furthermore, all four women were able to make the necessary shift from feeling they must put others first at the expense of their health to purposely taking care of themselves. This is not an easy task for low-income women with cancer, when resources are limited especially in a society that has imposed on them the posture of servitude.

Nevertheless, there is a difference in the severity of the cancer impact between Maria and the other three women interviewed. This difference is composed of both fear and physical side effects.

Whereas they speak of anxiety and fear, Maria speaks of fear and terror during her chemotherapy treatments that is comparable to one being tortured. Recalling her thoughts:

> Will I die on the elevator? Will I die while I wait for the taxi? In the cab she would dread the thought of dying there. At home she felt like she was drowning in fear because she was alone. . . . The fear was always waiting for her, torturing her by day and invading her nights with dreams of mutilated, dismembered bodies.

It was a horrendous metaphoric gasp that lasted long after treatment.

Chemotherapy weakened Maria for a prolonged period, far beyond the time it took Clare, Diane, and Lucia to physically recover from surgery. Unlike them, Maria was unable to return to work that first year. As a result, her isolation deepened and her financial devastation forced her first to seek General Assistance from welfare, and later SSI. Had she known of a support group, she would not have had the physical strength or energy to go. And, presentable clothes were unaffordable as she experienced major weight gain and other changes in her appearance: "I looked like someone with cushions. I had this big moon face and exaggerated dowager's hump. . . . My energy was close to zero." Occasionally, while she was walking down the street, a stranger would raise his voice to her without provocation, calling her a "fat pig," or worse.

Fortunately for Maria, no matter how she appeared to the world, or how discouraged she felt about her loss of energy, she still loved her life enough to believe it was worth living. The work she had done in therapy toward gaining a sense of self and self-acceptance saw her through, as she stated in her interview:

So, this business of gaining a sense of self and empowerment, it's very, very central, I think, to living. I think it's the
most important thing there is, and I got it from therapy. . . .
With other challenges earlier in my life, it was all yang
energy. It was just: I have to do this and I will *do it*. You can
only hold up so long with that kind of an attitude, that kind
of force. It won't take care of your life. But the idea of a
sense of self and nurturing the self and empowering your-
self, then that's good energy for your life. That's not just
hanging on in a crisis, but real strength.

This brings us to the concept of nurturing oneself throughout
the cancer experience, which can often be totally different from
what a low-income woman has learned to do. It is also the
opposite of the medical metaphor of waging war on cancer.
Although surgery, chemotherapy, and radiation are thought to be
the physician's main arsenal of weaponry, Maria, and others like
her, show us an inner strength of self-healing that is sustained by
nurturing. Nurturing oneself also means nurturing the immune
system through any number of ways: hypnotherapy, homeopathy, acupuncture, supportive herbs, nutrition, vitamin supplements, music, massage, emotional support, and surrounding oneself by the sweet breezes, sights, and sounds of nature are some
of many from which to choose.

This is not meant to downplay the benefits of allopathic medicine but, instead, to see the benefits of integrating complementary methods of nurturing both body and spirit so we can as a
whole society go beyond seeing the body as a battleground and
move toward healing. Low-income women in particular need
this because in their lives many have had so little opportunity for
nurturing.

Maria, therefore, teaches us two important facts to remember
in understanding and assisting low-income women with cancer.
First, a low-income woman who must endure long-term chemo-

therapy can be expected to experience more extreme side effects for a longer period of time, making the impact of cancer greater and the aftermath more prolonged. Although many will do better in chemotherapy than Maria, they are quite likely to have greater fear and more isolation as a result of a profound loss of energy, physical strength, and stamina. This is in addition to the usual nausea, vomiting, hair loss, diminished immune function, and other traumas induced by cancer and its treatment.

Cancer is a disease of loss that robs a low-income woman of so much more than if she were middle class because she already has so little at the time of the initial onslaught. Even if she has strong emotional support, the absence of a financial safety net leaves her vulnerable to an impact so great that it is almost impossible for the middle-class mind-set to comprehend.

The second fact Maria teaches us is that the low-income women with cancer who present as apathetic or hopeless can be helped toward hopeful self-determination. When psychotherapy is not available or desirable from the client's point of view, we can still provide the fertile conditions of nurturing for a strong sense of self to take root and grow. It may not be strong at first, but there is hope for deep healing.

We as workers can provide dynamic listening, support, validation, space for decision making, and that all-important acceptance. These nutrients must stem from respect for our client, from seeing her as an equal, competent person with her own wisdom, if she is to blossom into her own strong, nurturing sense of self. Therein lies her ability to spring from passive to proactive, from battle scarred to healing. How then, can we offer less?

Chapter 6

Case Management

One of the most important things we need to remember is that people who have cancer are on a roller coaster. One day they receive bad news, the next day good news. Each test result has momentous impact, as does every word the doctor speaks. A patient can experience hope and despair within a five-minute time frame—not just once, but over and over. This cannot be avoided. With each case, new information comes to light all during the course of treatment of this complicated disease. Cancer is an emotional batterer. For this reason, continuity and stability are both basic and necessary in promoting recovery.

When a middle-class woman develops cancer, much of her support is already in place or within reach. She already has transportation, groceries, some nutritional knowledge, cash on hand, credit, a secure place to live, and family members who share responsibilities. If she needs a wig, or someone to help with the housework, she can probably fit it into the budget. Likewise, her family members have the same kinds of basic needs already met so they are in a position to provide both practical and emotional support, although it may not be enough. When it isn't, the middle-class woman usually has enough sense of self-esteem, self, and sense of entitlement to utilize community resources such as support groups, a cancer library, and alternative supportive therapies. She does not expect the mainstream community to turn her away. Therefore, she probably has no need for a case manager.

By contrast, the low-income woman's life lacks most of the assets that her middle-class counterpart can rely on to provide continuity and stability in an ongoing crisis. Since I discuss the low-income woman's position in society in other parts of this book, there is no need to provide further details here. Suffice it to say that she is financially and sometimes emotionally insecure. Her family is less apt to give her strong support because they too have less than they need. Moreover, support outside the family may be almost nonexistent. Worst of all, the low-income woman is predisposed to being in the position of having no one, other than her doctor, who can or will say to her, "No matter what happens, I will see you through this." And this is what makes the role of case manager so crucial.

"I'm (or we're) going to help you through this," are the first words a low-income cancer patient needs to hear from her social worker. She needs to know she has emotional as well as practical support—that someone will listen. This is particularly important during the first few months following diagnosis before there has been an opportunity to connect with a support group. This will help offset the shock and sense of doom the low-income woman with cancer may be experiencing at that time. She also needs to know that she has someone to advocate for her anytime she might need it, and that it is all right to ask for help.

Naturally, the psychosocial assessment will provide the baseline for ongoing assistance. Attention to immediate basic needs should be preeminent. "Do you have enough groceries?" is an important question. Transportation to medical appointments and child care are among the problems she may be worrying about. Always ask her what she needs. Later, access to nutritional information and support groups can be discussed.

Physical weakness and fear are likely to be major barriers. Consider the one-time technique used by Maria's therapist that enabled her to actively fight the cancer. Helping the client to find ways to externalize her fear can make a significant difference in her recovery.

With your client's permission, meet separately with her family at least once to help them with questions, fears, or anything else that may prevent them from giving her their full support. Solicit their specific assistance with practical help such as cooking and laundry. Each family member will be able to think of ways to help. Involving the family will be instrumental in diminishing the sense of helplessness that cancer imposes.

Remember that people who are living with someone who is in an ongoing crisis do not always think of the obvious ways to help. A person who has never been in chemotherapy has no idea how much simple things, such as helping with the cleaning, can make a difference. People need to be told these things. Even if they are already supportive, they need to know how important that support is.

As discussed elsewhere in this book, it is coping with cancer— the ability to swing into action—that can make the difference in recovery. As the mind-body connection is brought into ever sharper focus through studies and becomes recognized as essential to the healing process, we can look forward to a more holistic approach in oncology.

Hopefully, the day will soon arrive when every cancer patient, particularly the low-income woman, will be routinely seen by both an oncologist and a social worker.

Chapter 7

Support Group Planning

> The oppressed, who have been shaped by the death-affirm-
> ing climate of oppression, must find through their struggle
> the way to live—affirming humanization . . . because their
> situation has reduced them to things. (Friere, 1990, p. 55)

For a number of years, middle-class women with cancer have
had the benefits of support groups. Unfortunately, we cannot say
the same for low-income women, and since support groups are
relatively unusual for poor women, we need to consider certain
dynamics in order to anticipate problems that may arise and to
ensure the success of such groups. We need first to be aware of the
stresses experienced as a result of being a woman who has cancer
and who also has been experiencing oppression over a long period
of time, particularly when she happens to be a woman of color.
This is of utmost importance because oppression and stress appear
to suppress the immune system.

Further, we need also to examine the dynamics of group composition in preparing the way for members to share information
and experiences and to form strong, supportive bonds. "On a
mental level, *knowledge* dispels fear, while on an emotional
level, *love* works every time" (Gawler, 1987, p. 147).

Group support is even more important for a woman in poverty
than for her middle-class counterpart because:

> The more unfortunate the plight or the greater the distress,
> the more threatened, uncomfortable, and rejecting other
> people tend to become. Those most in need of formal sup-
> port are less likely to receive it. (Northern, 1990, p. 15)

And, once a malignancy develops:

> Economic status is a factor in survival. After controlling for primary care factors and other variables, the poorer had worse survival than the patients who were in a higher socio-economic class. (Anderson, 1986, p. 73)

Then there is the stigma of having cancer. That is to say, society's attitudes tend toward oppression:

> The disease . . . is felt to be obscene in the original meaning of that word: ill-omened, abominable, repugnant to the senses . . . is viewed by some as the embodiment of repressed emotional or even violent feelings: this belief holds that the patient is somehow responsible for the disease—that it is the patient's failure of expressiveness which condemns him [her]. (McFate, 1979, p. 59)

This can have a damaging effect:

> For all individuals, self-esteem is built upon feelings of being accepted and acceptable. Cancer's "silent stigma" and its crippling psychosocial effects are a reality . . . financial worries, concerns about becoming a burden or a "vegetable," feelings of guilt and being punished . . . all have surfaced. (Eisman and Pumphrey, 1979, p. 219)

Furthermore:

> Stigmatization makes the individual seem less than human, allows others to explain her difficulties as a result of her inferiority, and to exercise discrimination in ways that effectively reduce her life chances . . . [and] self-derogation is likely. (Belle, 1982, p. 96)

Both Cassileth and Belle's above descriptions are surely intensified for any woman who has had to apply for welfare.

In addition, women, especially poor women, have multiple roles that others expect them to maintain. Low-income women have no financial resources to pay extra for help with domestic services, transportation, and other indirect expenses such as special diet foods, wigs, and over-the-counter medicines, appliances, and comfort aids while they are in treatment. To say they have considerable discomfort is an understatement. They are accustomed to giving priority to the needs of others and bringing order to others' lives, but they are now faced with a chaotic disease that may present an even greater threat to their lives if they continue to put other people ahead of their own healing.

Although many may not seem to be able to make the transition of giving their own lives first priority, at least not right away or to a great degree, it is crucial for a group facilitator to be aware of the importance of a woman who has cancer to be able to really focus on coping. The result, at best, can be spontaneous remission, which Dr. Siegel calls "self-induced healing." He tells his cancer patients, "Go to the mirror. Look in it, and save the person you see there" (Siegel, 1989, p. 199).

Although this may not be a physical, literal possibility for every individual:

> In a study of women with metastatic breast cancer, in which women were randomly assigned to intervention and control conditions, Siegal, Bloom, Kraemer, and Gottheil (1989) found at the ten-year follow-up that women who had participated in groups lived longer than women in the control condition. (Schopler and Galinsky, 1993, p. 198)

However, success may not take place unless the facilitator highly respects and values each group member, is aware of and is sensitive to cultural differences, and always remembers that "supportive assistance should complement the patient's (and/or client's) internal resources and life situation rather than interfere with them" (Stoll, 1979, p. 141). We cannot allow middle-class values to dominate. Instead, we need to remember "any assimilative process is the outcome of some form of dominance relation" (Menchaca, 1988, p. 228).

Lum further illustrates the concept of respect for low-income support group members:

> Social work must be aware of societal influences on its values and ethics. A middle-class social worker and a ghetto resident may respond to different physical, economic, and cultural realities. . . . Unlike third world thought, Western knowledge theory emphasizes the freedom and independence of the individual . . . [there is] a reliance on verbal exchange and analysis. Minority knowledge theory, on the other hand, emphasizes the individual's membership and functioning within the collective family, community, and ethnic group. Knowledge theory involves ethnic helpers, customs, and cosmic forces in the process. (Lum, 1986, pp. 25-26)

Although ethnic groups are each unique, their response to health issues can be similar. We see this in a study of breast cancer screening behaviors and attitudes: "In general, similar patterns of association were observed across racial/ethnic groups" (Vernon et al., 1992, p. 173).

Probably the most important concern in an ethnically mixed membership is to avoid a *"psychological minority* [which] refers to a disproportionate decrease in an individual's sense of security and control" (Davis, 1980, p. 77). That is, every member must be given as much warmth, acceptance, and attention as the next, regardless.

And, to further increase success, we need to be aware that:

> The effectiveness of any group is determined partially by the particular attributes or characteristics that each individual brings to the group. Attributes are of two kinds: "descriptive" such as age, sex, marital status, etc. and "behavioral" attrib-

utes, which indicate how an individual interacts with others, [and which] are much better predictors of an individual's behavior in a group. Effective groups tend to have interactive, compatible, and responsive members. Interactive members like each other. Responsive members are interested in helping each other. (Bertcher, 1971, p. 187)

This brings us to the question of how best to select group members. We may need a systematic, theoretical framework such as Schultz's theory of Fundamental Interpersonal Relations Orientations (FIRO).

Schultz states that each person has the need to establish satisfactory relationships with others in three basic interpersonal needs areas—affection, control, and inclusion. [and that] Interchange compatibility is characterized by the degree to which people have a desire for affection, control, or inclusion. Reciprocal compatibility measures the degree a person wants to receive the behavior expressed by another, and vice versa, in any need area. (Shalinsky, 1967, p. 42)

According to Schultz, the inclusion, control, and affection phases can be seen as parallel with the needs of childhood, adolescence, and adulthood, respectively. In fact, "This postulate states that every interpersonal relation follows the same course of development and resolution" (Schultz, 1950, p. 168). The inclusion phase is finding out where one fits in, learning that one won't be ignored, and establishing boundaries: How involved do I want to be? In the control phase, there is anxiety over too much or too little control. This is where struggle for leadership may take place. The affection phase is a time of emotional integration, jealousy, pairing, personal hostility, and anxiety over intimacy. "All three problem areas are always present but not of equal salience" (Schultz, 1950, pp. 168-171).

It follows that, if a group is high on inclusion compatibility, members will be most compatible during the initial stages; if the group is high on control compatibility, members will be most cooperative during the middle stages; if the group is high on affection compatibility, members will be most compatible prior to the termination phase. And, most important, "For the longer term groups which reach the affection phase, how well people fit together with regard to affection should be central" (Schultz, 1950, p. 179). Although we may find some mixing will be suitable, we are still in a better position to avoid pitfalls and to enhance cohesiveness, which is a major, necessary component of this kind of group.

The positive results of planning and paying attention to the psychosocial dynamics can be realized far beyond expectations when empowerment is the dominant theme. "[T]he power of interpersonal relations and social well-being that the small group can make possible in the process of healing and sustaining health has been growing in recognition" (Schopler and Galinsky, 1990, p. 4).

Although we can see that oppression in any form may bring on stress that is destructive enough to play a role in the development of cancer, there also is hope in coping through group support:

> Whether the course of cancer results in recovery or death, it is possible to help people preserve their self-respect and maximize their opportunities to control those aspects of their lives which have importance for them. Even in the terminal stage people can be helped to participate in the planning for themselves, or others such as minor children, [and] elderly. (Domanski et al., 1979, p. 106)

In summary:

> . . . while it is true socioeconomic status may not necessarily determine how well a woman faces her cancer, how well she survives it, or how well she understands it, poverty is a powerful predictor of late diagnosis, poor treatment, and

high mortality. Women in this country are disproportion-ately poor; women of color are the most disproportionately poor. The recent mobilization of women . . . must, there-fore, actively incorporate poverty and the interaction of racism, sexism, and poverty as primary focus, since poverty so clearly influences women's experience of disease and their expectations of survival. (Hardisty and Leopold, 1992, p. 8)

Although class issues are seldom mentioned when discussing the question of why low-income women rarely join support groups, we would do well to understand that when a woman is poor, she has been oppressed. How much she has been oppressed may depend on the number of factors, such as race, poverty, and body size, that prevent her from being a respected member of society. But, no matter what the degree of oppression, it is the dual presence of oppression and cancer that various low-income women have in common. Therefore, assuming there is no lan-guage barrier, a support group of the same economic class of women with cancer has the potential for success even when they are of different ethnic backgrounds, providing that the members tend to be warm people.

The exception might be women who have been poor all their lives but yet have managed to acquire higher education. An unrecognized minority, these may have the greatest emotional discomfort because they must constantly straddle two worlds. Some, of course, are able to integrate fully into the middle class.

Equally important to group members being able to relate to each other is the willingness and ability of the facilitator to give each member as much warmth and acceptance and attention as the next. Sensitivity is the offspring of compassion.

One factor that is rarely considered carefully enough, even in middle-class cancer groups, is the stage at the time of diagnosis, or how advanced any particular group member's cancer is. Many a newly diagnosed woman has been frightened away from a support group when she hears the stories of women with metastasis or of others with a poor prognosis. This can also lead to depression and should be avoided, if at all possible.

Also, it is not usually a good idea to include family and friends in the same group with cancer patients. People who are close to each other often will try to protect one another's feelings, making it difficult for the woman with cancer to speak freely. She may already be guarding her family's feelings at home. This is her time to let go of that burden. Support groups for families and friends are both useful and important, but they should be separate for best results. It can also be very helpful for the social worker to meet with a client and her family. However, that should not replace a support group. It would be a disservice to the client.

Chapter 8

Three Community Models

THE CHARLOTTE MAXWELL COMPLEMENTARY CLINIC (CMCC)

The Charlotte Maxwell Complementary Clinic is named in honor of Charlotte Maxwell who died of ovarian cancer. She was committed to the idea of making complementary forms of care available to women with cancer who ordinarily can't afford to pay for them and might not know about them.

Licensed by the state of California, this clinic provides low-income women with modalities to help them deal with cancer and the side effects of treatment. These modalities include acupuncture, massage, visualization, homeopathy, and social work services. All services are free of charge. However, CMCC does require that each client has her own medical doctor outside the clinic.

The clinic's social work services include counseling concerning issues of cancer (not psychotherapy), crisis intervention, advocacy, case management, and resource referral with support groups soon to be implemented. Recently, CMCC has become a field training agency for undergraduate and graduate social work students. CMCC fully supports the entire spectrum of client choice, regarding treatment as well as lifestyle changes.

"Charlotte's Web," the client-created newsletter, is a significant resource that reduces stress and isolation. Its articles and poems inform, enlighten, and comfort as they weave together the threads of the cancer journey. Sometimes, clients are interviewed, with each spinning her own unique story that somehow always resonates with the experience of other low-income women with cancer. Most important, this gentle, strong "web" connects clients so that to-gether they are a cohesive, supportive community—women with a voice.

Staff and volunteers are caring and nonjudgmental, as well as respectful of differences: class, race, culture, sexual preference, spiritual beliefs, and body size. The emotional environment is warm, egalitarian, and inclusive. Furthermore, workers will do everything possible to prevent a woman from blaming herself for her cancer. With the exact cause(s) of cancer unknown, it is believed there are numerous contributing factors such as poverty, racism, and environmental poisons.

CMCC has been rapidly expanding in response to community needs. It began in 1991 as a four-hour, Saturday operation and is now open to approximately sixty-five clients for twelve weekend hours, requiring the support of about one-hundred volunteers, two social work interns, and three paid part-time positions.

Financial support is provided by private donations and grants. Recently, a grant has been awarded by the Breast Cancer Research Program to fund a study regarding the efficacy of a three-day retreat for low-income women with breast cancer.

Pioneering in spirit and praised by both its clients and the surrounding community, CMCC was presented with a letter of commendation by Shirley Dean, Mayor of Berkeley.

For more information, call or write:

Charlotte Maxwell Complementary Clinic
5346 College Avenue
Oakland, CA 94618
(510) 601-7660

THE WOMEN'S CANCER RESOURCE CENTER

The Women's Cancer Resource Center (WCRC) is a haven for women who have cancer. Its purpose is to empower these women through providing critically needed services at no charge in the areas of information, support, and advocacy. It is funded by sources such as foundation grants and private donations. WCRC serves a spectrum of women, including lesbians, women of color, non-English speaking women, older women and disabled women as well.

The center was founded in 1986 by a small group of lesbian cancer survivors possessing organizational skills, who were both startled and angered by the lack of support services for women with cancer. At that time, WCRC consisted of a single telephone in someone's living room and just enough volunteers to answer it. Responding to the ever-growing needs of the community, the center now has over 120 volunteers, a board of directors, several committees, and a staff of five. It has provided services to more than 25,000 women.

Services include an information and referral hotline, support groups, a lending library of over 8,000 books, and an on-line medical data base along with medical textbooks and reference books. The librarian accepts nationwide requests for reference materials and on-line research packets on any particular kind of cancer with allopathic and/or alternative medicine information. Information is tailored specific to the requester regarding age, educational level, date of diagnosis, and stage of cancer.

Active in the community, WCRC helped form a coalition for promoting changes within the health care system to make it more responsive to women's needs. Offshoots of this coalition include quarterly meetings, cooperative political action, networking, a growing awareness of the services provided by the various agencies within the coalition, and an annual fundraising Women and Cancer Walk. Also, WCRC is an active member of the National Coalition of Feminist and Lesbian Cancer Projects.

Recognized both at home and nationally, WCRC was voted the Best Community Organization in the 1993 Readers Poll in *Express,* a Berkeley newspaper. It has been mentioned in *The New York*

Times, the *Village Voice,* the *MacNeil-Lehrer News Report,* ABC *Evening News,* and *Ms. Magazine.*

Again, the Women's Cancer Resource Center is a model for serving and empowering women who have cancer. It has assisted the development of similar projects around the country. For information on how to form a resource center for women with cancer, call or write to:

Diane Estrin, Executive Director
Women's Cancer Resource Center
3023 Shattuck Avenue
Berkeley, California 94705
(510) 548-9272

BREAST CANCER ACTION (BCA)

Breast Cancer Action is a grassroots organization of breast cancer survivors and their supporters. It publishes an informative bimonthly newsletter and is actively dedicated to the prevention and cure of breast cancer.

Politically effective, BCA was the driving force that provided the choice to allocate money for breast cancer research on federal income tax forms. In addition, BCA meets with and coordinates its efforts with other individuals and groups, including researchers and environmentalists. We can expect to hear much more about this group of activists in the future.

A nonprofit organization, Breast Cancer Action is funded in part by the Junior League of San Francisco, as well as through donations. BCA welcomes the support of those who want to join in the fight against breast cancer. Although subscribers to the BCA newsletter are expected to contribute, no one is turned away for lack of funds.

For more information, contact:

Barbara A. Brenner, Executive Director
Breast Cancer Action
55 New Montgomery Street
San Francisco, Ca 94105
(415) 243-9301

Chapter 9

Prevention and Social Work: An Environmental Approach

Cancer is the leading cause of death among women ages thirty-five to fifty-four. (Arditte and Schreiber, 1993, p. 235)

Since 1971, when President Nixon first declared war on cancer, the United States has spent one trillion dollars—a sum nearly a third as large as the national debt—on cancer research and treatment. Despite this money, the number of cases and the number of deaths from the disease rise inexorably every year. (Brady, 1991a, pp. 8-9)*

Since this declaration, former President Nixon's own wife, Patricia, died of cancer, and more recently, President Clinton's mother has also succumbed to this disease.

Where is the cure we were promised so long ago? Why does the media keep implying great strides are being made and we must remain hopeful, while more and more of the people we love are dying all around us? Where is cancer on the list of priorities in this country?

Limping into the twenty-first century without a cure, Western medicine provides weapons such as surgeries that maim, drugs that destroy healthy cells along with tumor cells, and radiation that can itself cause new malignancies.

---

* Some material in this chapter has been quoted from Judy Brady, *1 in 3: Women with Cancer Confront an Epidemic,* © by Judy Brady. *1 in 3* is published by Cleis Press: 1-800-780-2279.

Disregarding that failure, emphasis is now being placed on behavior and early detection:

> Psychosocial and behavioral factors in human cancer affect both the risk of developing cancer and the length of survival once cancer has developed. . . . Cancer prevention programs depend heavily on . . . reducing smoking and alcohol intake, lowering dietary fat intake, [and] increasing dietary fiber. (DeVita, Hellman, and Rosenberg, 1989, p. 2204)

Naturally, this advice is beneficial. It makes sense to take care of our bodies in the hope that they will be healthy and last longer. Surely, nutrition is important, as is the avoidance of cigarette smoke.

However, IT IS NOT ENOUGH. "Even the most conservative scientists agree that approximately 80 percent of all cancers are in some way related to environmental factors" (Arditte and Schreiber, 1993, p. 233). It seems that if environmental factors had only to do with healthy lifestyles—that is, if they were within the control of the individual—people who take care of their bodies would not get cancer. There has to be some factor that exists which is beyond the individual's control.

> Two years ago, at the age of thirty-nine, I was diagnosed with breast cancer. I was profoundly shocked. I had been healthy and vigorous all my life, my parents are healthy and vigorous septuagenarians, and there is no noteworthy history of cancer in my extended family. (Seventy-five percent of women diagnosed with breast cancer have no family history of the disease and no other known risk factors) . . . the bugs that laid others low rarely got me. I saw myself as relentlessly healthy and quietly relished my hardiness, which I attributed to good

genes, decent health habits, and a characterological forti-
tude. (Kofron, 1993, p. 35)*

Kofron goes on to say, "There is nothing unique about my experience" (p. 36).

There is also nothing new or unique about fat being present in
the human body and in the human diet—it has been with us for
centuries. Cancer, on the other hand, seems to be a twentieth-
century disease. When we compare these two time frames, it
does not seem likely that fat alone would be the key ingredient in
certain kinds of cancer. Nonetheless, research shows a direct
association:

> "The results are too consistent to believe that the association
> is indirect," says Maureen Henderson, an epidemiologist at
> the Fred Hutchinson Cancer Research Center in Seattle.
> "When it comes to the breast cancer connection," she says
> flatly, "I'm sure of it." (Wallas, 1991, p. 50)

What is it that makes previously benign fat so lethal in this century?

Dr. Mary S. Wolf conducted the New York University Women's
Health Study of 14,290 women between 1985 and 1991 and found
higher levels of PCB (polychlorinated biphenyls) and DDE (the
end product of DDT) in breast cancer patients. Dr. Wolf summa-
rizes her findings: "Given the widespread dissemination of organo-
chlorine insecticides in the environment and the food chain, the
implications are far-reaching for public health worldwide"
(McGregor, 1993, pp. 7-11). "Although banned in the United
States since 1972, DDT persists in the soil and accumulates in the
fat tissues of animals and humans" (Tanne, 1993, p. 57). There we
have it. It is not the fat per se, but rather, it is the pesticide
accumulation in the fat that is the lethal ingredient.

---

*Quotations cited Kofron, 1993 are from "The Language of Cancer," by Emily
E. Kofron. This article first appeared in the *Family Therapy Networker* and is
copied here with permission.

Unfortunately, or perhaps purposefully, the American Cancer Society (ACS) and the National Cancer Institute (NCI) seem to play a major role in skewing public opinion toward blaming the victim.

> Public education campaigns of cancer establishments such as the ACS and the NCI focus almost exclusively on individual habit (diet, smoking, sunbathing, and breast self-exams) when addressing cancer prevention. This analysis never acknowledges that personal habits are themselves social constructions. But more importantly, an emphasis on life-style obscures the role of environmental hazards that are beyond personal choice. (Steingraber, 1991, p. 41)

One tragic result is the rose-colored blindness we have in our perception of the health of American babies:

> These days babies are born with compromised immune systems; they have dioxin and a veritable arsenal of other chemicals stored in their bodies before they take their first breath. The breast milk they drink—produced in that tissue which so readily responds to ionizing radiation—is full of alien substances. Children eat food laden with pesticides and chemical additives. They breathe car exhaust. They live in the shadow of nuclear plants and dumps and in plastics factories and other places that expose them to carcinogens, known and unknown. The United States is a dangerous place to live.
>
> When we had a country without this kind of pollution, the cancer rate was low; with this kind of pollution, the cancer is high (Brady, 1991a, p. 9).

Furthermore, the New York Coalition for Alternatives to Pesticides (NYCAP) (1993) tells us:

> When a teacher made too ill to work by pesticides describes how her kindergarten children would get sick like clock-

work the day after the spraying, you realize that we are slowly poisoning the future generations . . . (although substitutes for cancer-causing and nerve-damaging pesticides are cost competitive and highly effective (p. 1). . . . [and] An epidemiological study published this January found a link between brain cancer in children and home pesticide use. (pp. 5-6)

According to Berger and Kelly (1993), "We are exposed to some 100,000 chemicals, many of them . . . known to cause biological harm" but are still "manufactured in large quantities and dispersed in our foods, the air we breathe, and the water we drink" (p. 53).

Even the *Merck Manual* admits to agents that "directly induce malignant transformation . . . and subsequent DNA damage" and then lists some, plus "ionizing radiation due to nuclear incidences and X-rays." It goes on to say: "Long-term exposure to occupational irradiation or to internally deposited thorium dioxide predisposes persons to develop angiosarcomas and acute nonlymphocytic leukemia (Berkow, 1987, pp. 1208-1209).

And where does the low-income woman find herself in all of this? Chances are she is living a short life next door to toxic waste:

Poor women and women of color die disproportionately from cancer, because they lack early and appropriate medical treatment, and are often in greater proximity to toxic waste dumps and other environmental carcinogens. (Kofron, 1993, p. 42)

Steingraber (1991) concurs:

. . . well-documented cancer clusters have been mapped in communities located near chemical factories, refineries, nuclear reactors, and pesticide-saturated farm fields. These are not randomly selected communities; they are, more often than not, poor and nonwhite. Of the 140,000 toxic waste dumps that have been identified in the United States, for example, 60 percent are located in Black or Hispanic neighborhoods. (p. 41)

The low-income woman, whatever her ethnic background, may not be aware of the danger to her and her family. She certainly can't afford to buy bottled water and organically grown food in order to arm herself with that healthy lifestyle we hear so much about. Also, life has taught her to have a sense of powerlessness, economically and politically.

Zinna, one such woman, a Native American, writes of her experience living "downwind" from Hanford, a nuclear complex in Washington state. Battered by her husband and then stricken by cancer, she had to deal with a society that blames its victims:

> In my frantic search for a means of survival for myself and my children, I turned to various social agencies for help. I found neither help nor encouragement. Rather, I was confronted with condemnation for being both poor and ill; I was a double failure. (Epperson, 1991, p. 92)

But her problems were just beginning. Besides cancer, Zinna developed lupus:

> [M]y body does not metabolize properly anymore . . . my spine continues to disintegrate . . . [there is] progression of weakness and fatigue . . . and multiple sclerosis like reactions to the sun . . .
>
> Of ten pregnancies, I have four surviving. All have degenerative spinal problems. (Epperson, 1991, p. 94)

Zinna goes on to describe her family's multiple health problems and then portrays attitudes that made her situation worse:

> Positive thinking groups insisted that I really wanted to be ill when I failed to think myself well. Religious groups

accused me of not trusting God when I failed to be miracu-
lously cured. Mental health agencies told me that I harbored
subconscious negative anger from my childhood because it
was proven that negative emotions cause cancer. And welfare seemed more interested in taking my children away
from me than in helping me raise them. With the "assistance" of those agencies, I felt useless and ashamed because
I could no longer hold a paying job. (Epperson, 1991, p. 94)

"Blaming the victim is a time-honored method of deflecting orga-
nized opposition and protecting a power base" (Brady, 1991b,
p. 28).

We live in a society where business and profits come first, and
people, particularly low-income women and their children, are low
on the list of priorities. "Eco-feminists, for example, have pointed
out the connections between sex-role socialization and ecology.
Current attitudes toward ecology have been shaped by a male ethic
that stresses disconnectedness, hierarchy, and power over the
world" (Berger and Kelly, 1993, p. 524).

Consequently, "The incidence of certain cancers has grown dra-
matically, yet there seems to be a bewildering unwillingness to
examine and act upon the obvious link to environmental toxins"
(Kofron, 1993, p. 36).

Instead, we are consistently being told the chemicals and radioactive materials that cause cancer in laboratory animals are used in
such small amounts in products for humans so as to be rendered
harmless. Telling the public that proven carcinogens are harmless is
an outright lie. Implying they are not cumulative is another lie. We
are already inundated with nuclear damage, as shown in the *Townsend Letter for Doctors:*

Recent studies now suggest that one hitherto neglected factor is the unexpectedly severe biological action of radioactive
releases from aging nuclear reactors into the milk and water

supplies of major metropolitan areas . . . [which are] a secondary insult to the immune systems initially damaged by the fallout from atmospheric bomb tests in the period extending roughly from 1944 to 1965, equivalent to some 40,000 Hiroshima bombs . . .

The unexpectedly large effects produced by inhaled or ingested nuclear fission products on the immune system, leading to premature birth, to low birth weight, and renewed rises in infectious diseases and cancer . . . [also includes] the increased mutation rate of microorganisms, which is greater at low rather than high dose rates. (Null, Sternglass, and Gould, 1993, p. 812)

Furthermore,

Recent articles in *Science* delineate the enormous public health crisis set off by the increasing resistance to antibiotics of those mutating microorganisms responsible for AIDS, tuberculosis, shigellosis, salmonella, toxic shock syndrome, Lyme disease and many other newly emerging and old infections. Thus, in addition to causing immune deficiency, fission products would accelerate the mutation rate of microorganisms leading to new epidemics on a worldwide basis, and the new strains would be far more deadly. (Null, Sternglass, and Gould, 1993, p. 813)

This shocking evidence leaves us wondering why physicians, when they question cancer patients about their medical histories and lifestyles, do not ask about radiation, pesticide, and other chemical exposures: " . . . regardless of any individual oncologist's dedication, in a health care-for-profit system, cancer is the goose that lays the golden egg." In 1991 a total of $750,000,000 was spent on chemotherapy drugs in the United States. And every year we can expect costs to rise (Brady, 1991b, pp. 25-26). The prescription drug industry is very lucrative and powerful.

Continuing our look at money and power, when we read *The Cancer Industry*, we find the behind-the-scene driving power of the Memorial Sloan-Kettering Cancer Center (MSKCC):

> An analysis of the leadership of the world's largest private cancer center shows that those men and women with a vested interest in the cancer problem control the direction of research.
>
> The board of overseers . . . is composed of fifty-two individuals. Only four of these are medical doctors and three others are PhDs . . .
>
> The industry that stands to gain the most from cancer research is the pharmaceutical business. This industry in particular has great influence on the MSKCC board . . .
>
> . . . seventeen overseers—or 32.7 percent—are rather closely tied to large polluting industries, especially those connected to oil, chemicals, and automobiles . . .
>
> The other main vested interest of the overseers is in corporate investments. Many of these men and women are bankers, stockbrokers, and venture capitalists . . . eighteen out of fifty-two or 36 percent are professional investors or persons closely associated . . . the chairman of the board, Laurance S. Rockefeller . . . is a self-described capitalist. (Moss, 1989, pp. 441, 445, 446)

Where, we must ask, are the government agencies to protect us, and what are they doing about this crisis? Listed under "Government Agencies" are thirteen such agencies, their locations, telephone numbers, and functions, according to the *Cancer-Prevention Resource Directory*, United States Department of Health and Human Services, Public Health Service, and National Institutes of Health.

Since it is difficult, if at all possible, to recall any time in recent years when any of these agencies have communicated with the American public, we do not know if they have been making efforts to protect public health or not. If they have, the evidence uncovered in this book leads us to believe that they have either failed or sold out. Furthermore, in the interest of real cancer prevention, we can challenge them publicly to explain what they have been doing while people continue to die of cancer in even greater numbers. To whom are they bound in probity to be accountable, if not the American people?

Are there no laws to protect us? Isn't there something called the Delaney Clause? Yes, but even that is in jeopardy.

The Delaney Clause (Section 409 of the Federal Food and Drug and Cosmetic Act of 1958, authored by Congressman James Delaney, Dem., New York) prohibits the Federal Drug Administration (FDA) approval of any food additive found to cause cancer in humans or animals.

However, the FDA and the United States Department of Agriculture (USDA) are squeezed between the Delaney Clause and the pesticide industry. As a result, they:

> asked the National Academy of Sciences to examine the "zero-tolerance" provisions of the Delaney Clause, which in 1965 determined that improved measuring techniques allowed the detection of very small amounts of chemical residues, so zero would not be found. (Of course zero would be found if the toxic chemicals were banned entirely, but the Academy did not discuss that politically incorrect alternative.) (NYCAP, 1993, pp. 5-6)

The actions that followed may well be viewed in retrospect as the greatest atrocity in American history because the end result is death unlimited: "On April 13, 1966, the two agencies began establishing allowable levels ('tolerances') of cancer-causing pesticides," totally disregarding the mounting scientific evidence that points to the devastating impact of cumulative toxins (NYCAP, 1993, p. 6).

Unlike the Delaney Clause Section 409 which prohibits cancer-causing chemicals, Section 408 allows officials to weigh the value of abundant cheap food against a few thousand deaths and conclude those deaths have a negligible value. "In short, twenty-eight pesticides cause 20,700 deaths per year." The Delaney Clause is not a scientific anachronism—it is more valid now than in 1958. Cancer statistics are rising and our loved ones are among them. This demonstrates the profit-before-people priorities of American business (NYCAP, 1993, p. 6).

Definitely, there is a role for social work—an important one that has global implications in this crisis. Besides understanding more deeply and delivering services to low-income women who have cancer, it is crucial that we take a stand against environmental toxins. In so doing, we will best serve the low-income woman, and ourselves as well, through the real prevention of cancer. "The ability of humans to survive ecological disruptions will depend on the development of a new global ethic, one that respects ecological values" (Berger and Kelly, 1993, p. 523).

Berger and Kelly have set forth for us an important Ecological Credo that warrants our adoption. It is quoted, according to the National Association of Social Workers Journal, in Chapter 11.

Beyond that, to social workers and to others who care, this is a call to action.

Onward.

Chapter 10

Government Agencies

Cancer Control Science Program
National Cancer Institute
National Institutes of Health
Bethesda, MD 20892-4200
(301) 427-8771

Seeks to ensure that research results are effectively applied in a timely manner to the nation's cancer control problems.

Center for Health Promotion and Education
Centers for Disease Control
Building 1 South, Room SSB249
1600 Clifton Road, NE
Atlanta, GA 30333
(404) 329-3492

Prevention Programs:

1. Technical assistance to states and local health departments to track risk factor conditions in the population
2. Behavioral risk factor surveillance system and survey
3. School health education evaluation project

Taken from the *Cancer Prevention-Resource Directory* of the U.S. Department of Health and Human Services, Public Health Service, and National Institutes of Health, pp. 13-16.

Clearinghouse on Health Indexes
National Center for Health Statistics
Division of Epidemiology and Health Promotion
3700 East-West Highway, Room 2-27
Hyattsville, MD 20782
(301) 436-7035

Provides informational assistance to develop health measures to health researchers, administrators, and planners.

Clearinghouse for Occupational Safety and Health Information
National Institute for Occupational Safety and Health
Technical Information Branch
4676 Columbia Parkway
Cincinnati, OH 45226
(513) 684-8326

Supplies information (technical) to the Institute for Occupational Safety and Health research programs and others on request.

Consumer Product Safety Commission
Washington, DC 20207
(301) 492-6800
(800) 638-2772 (hotline)

An independent federal regulatory agency with jurisdiction over consumer products used in and around home, it sets standards and conducts information programs on potentially hazardous products including carcinogens. Single copies of printed materials are available—a free service.

Division of Cancer Prevention and Control
National Cancer Institute
National Institutes of Health
Bethesda, MD 20892-4200
(301) 496-6616

Plans and conducts basic and applied research programs aimed at reducing cancer incidence, morbidity, and mortality. Plans, directs, and coordinates support of research on cancer prevention and control at centers and community hospitals.

Food and Nutrition Information Center
U.S. Department of Agriculture
National Agricultural Library Building—Room 304
Beltsville, MD 20705
(301) 344-3719

Provides information to professionals on nutrition education and food service management.

Information Projects Branch
National Cancer Institute
National Institutes of Health
Bethesda, MD 20892-4200
(301) 496-6792

Develops materials and programs in response to cancer-related needs and concerns of the general public, health professionals, and cancer patients and their families.

National Audiovisual Center
National Archives
8700 Edgeworth Drive
Capital Heights, MD 20743-3701
(301) 763-1896
(301) 763-4385 (TDD)

Distributes over 8,000 programs on 600 topics including cancer and the environment, breast cancer, cancer detection, and smoking. The price range is $50 to $350.

National Toxicology Program
National Institute of Environmental Health Sciences
M.D. B2-04, Box 12233
Research Triangle Park, NC 27709
(919) 541-3991

Develops and disseminates scientific information regarding potentially hazardous chemicals, including those that can contribute to cancer. Also coordinates research conducted by four agencies of the Department of Health and Human Services. Provides free technical reports for scientists and the general public.

Office of Cancer Communications
National Cancer Institute
National Institutes of Health
Bethesda, MD 20892-4200
(301) 496-6631

Provides information on all aspects of the cancer problem to physicians, scientists, educators, Congress, the executive branch, media, and the public.

Public Distribution Office
Occupational Safety and Health Administration
U.S. Department of Labor
200 Constitution Avenue, NW—Room S4203
Washington, DC 20210
(202) 523-9667

Responds to inquiries about a limited number of job-related carcinogens and toxic substances—a free service.

Public Information Center
Environmental Protection Agency
820 Quincy Street, NW
Washington, DC 20011
(202) 829-3535

Provides materials on such topics as hazardous wastes, the school asbestos project, air and water pollution, pesticides, and drinking water.

Reports and Inquiries Branch
National Cancer Institute
National Institutes of Health
Bethesda, MD 20892-4200
(301) 496-6631

Responds to questions from the press and public about prevention, early detection, and treatment of cancer.

Chapter 11

Ecological Credo for Social Workers

Raymond M. Berger and James J. Kelly

1. Social work is concerned not only with the interactions between people and their social environments, but with the full range of interconnectedness among all systems within Earth's biosphere.
2. Social work promotes self-determination and respect for individuals within the context of individual and community respect for nature. Self-respect and respect for nature are inseparable.
3. Social work believes in global equality, that is, in the right of all people of the world to share equally in Earth's bounty. It recognizes that global harmony cannot exist when a minority of people in developed nations consume a disproportionate share of global resources.
4. Social work seeks the establishment of social and economic policies that promote human welfare. Human welfare is understood to include not only short-term needs for consumption but also the needs of future generations. Therefore, social work supports only those social and economic policies that promote sustainable use of Earth's resources.

Originally published in *Social Work,* journal of the National Association of Social Workers, September 1993, Volume 38, Number 5, pp. 524-525. Reprinted with permission.

5. Social work has the responsibility to promote social, political, and economic systems that respect the integrity of the biosphere. This support extends to new means of economic, social, and political organization that will reverse current practices of ecological damage and resource depletion.

6. Social work is confident of the integrity of the natural ecosystem. At the same time, social work acknowledges the carrying capacity of the biosphere and respects the limits of that capacity.

7. Social work values the principle of diversity. The diversity of ecological niches and life forms that form the biosphere is reflected in the diverse races, ethnic groups, cultures, and values of people. Such diversity is valued for the resilience it brings to all systems.

8. Social work assumes a global and universal perspective. Humans are not separate from, nor superior to, other parts of the biosphere. Rather, humans are but one aspect of a vast universe in which every aspect is interconnected.

9. Social work promotes stewardship of the Earth's resources by its human inhabitants.

10. Social work acknowledges the obligation of its professionals to speak out when they have knowledge of damage to the environment that will adversely affect the quality or sustainability of life for current or future generations of living systems.

11. Social work believes that humans have the moral capacity to apply their intelligence and technology to create ecologically sound, humane, and sustainable lifestyles.

12. Social work believes in the essential goodness of people. The people of Earth will voluntarily live in harmony with Earth's resources when afforded the opportunity to assume ecologically responsible lifestyles.

Bibliography

American Psychiatric Association (1987). *Diagnostic and statistical manual of mental disorders,* third edition, revised. Washington, DC: American Psychiatric Association, pp. 247-251, 384-385.

Anderson, B.L. (Ed.). (1986). *Women with cancer.* New York: Springer-Verlag.

Arditte, R. and Schreiber, T. (1993). Killing us quietly: Cancer, the environment, and women. In M. Stocker, *Confronting cancer, constructing change: New perspectives on women and cancer.* Chicago, IL: Third Side Press, pp. 232-235.

Bacon, C., Renneker, R., and Cutler, M. (1952/1979). Psychosomatic survey of cancer of the breast. In B.R. Cassileth, *The cancer patient.* Philadelphia, PA: Lea and Febiger, pp. 453-460.

Bell, D. S. (1991). *The disease of a thousand names: CFIDS chronic fatigue/immune dysfunction syndrome.* Lyndonville, NY: Pollard Publications.

Belle, D. (Ed.). (1982). *Lives in stress.* Beverly Hills, CA: Sage.

Berger, R.M. and Kelly, J.J. (1993). Social work in the ecological crisis. *Social Work,* 38(5): pp. 505-648.

Berkow, R. (Ed.-in-chief). (1987). *The Merck manual of diagnosis and therapy,* edition 15. Rathway, NJ: Merck, Sharp, and Dome Research Laboratories.

Bertcher, H. and Maple, F. (1971). Elements and issues in group composition. San Francisco, CA: In P. Glasser, R. Sarri, and R. Vinter, *Individual change through small groups.* New York: Free Press, pp. 186-208.

Bracht, N.F. (1978). *Social work in health care: A guide to professional practice.* Binghamton, NY: The Haworth Press, Inc.

Brady, J. (1991a). Introduction. In Judith Brady, *1 in 3: Women with cancer confront an epidemic.* San Francisco, CA: Cleis Press, pp. 8-10.

Brady, J. (1991b). The goose and the golden egg. In Judith Brady, *1 in 3: Women with cancer confront an epidemic.* San Francisco, CA: Cleis Press, pp. 13-35.

Butrym, Z. and Horder, J. (1983). *Health, doctors and social workers.* London: Routledge and Kegan.

Cancer Prevention Resource Directory. U.S. Department of Health and Human Services, Public Health Service, and National Institutes of Health, pp. 13-16.

Cassileth, B.R. (1979). *The cancer patient.* Philadelphia, PA: Lea and Febiger.

Cassileth, B.R., Lusk, E.J., Walsh, P., Doyle, B., and Maier, M. (1989). The satisfaction and psychosocial status of patients during treatment for cancer. *Journal of Psychosocial Oncology,* 7(4): pp. 1-29.

Clare, A.W. and Corney, R.H. (Eds.). (1982). *Social work and primary health care.* New York: Academic Press.

Claymon, S. (1993). One more thing to watch out for. *Breast Cancer Action,* August (19): pp. 7-11.

Cohen, F. and Lazarus, N.S. (1979). Coping with stresses of illness. In G.C. Stone and F. Cohen, *Health psychology—A handbook*. San Francisco: Jossey Bass Publishers, pp. 217-254.

Cohn, K.H. (1989). Chemotherapy from an insider's perspective: Reflections seven years later. *Journal of Psychosocial Oncology*, 7(4): p. 131.

Cooper, C.L. (Ed.). (1984). *Psychosocial stress and cancer*. Chichester, England: John Wiley and Sons.

Davis, L. (1980). Racial balance—A psychological issue: A note to group workers. *Social Work with Groups*, 3(2): pp. 75-85.

Delgado, M. (1983). Activities and Hispanic groups: Issues and suggestions. In R. Middleman, *Activities and action in groupwork*. Binghamton, NY: The Haworth Press, Inc., pp. 85-95.

DeVita, V.T., Hellman, S., and Rosenberg, S.A. (Eds.). (1989). *Cancer principles and practice of oncology*. Philadelphia, PA: J.B. Lippincott.

Domanski, M., Lipiec, K., Rensel, S., and Sherwin, K. (1979). Comprehensive care of the chronically ill cancer patient: An inter-agency model. *Social Work in Health Care*, 5(1): pp. 57, 75-77, 106.

Eisman, S.H. and Pumphrey, J.B. (1979). Patient adaptation to terminal illness. In B.R. Cassileth, *The cancer patient*. Philadelphia, PA: Lea and Febiger, pp. 219-232.

Ell, K.O. and Nishimoto, R.H. (1989). Coping resources in adaptation to cancer: Socioeconomical and racial differences. *Social Service Review*, September: pp. 433-445.

Englisbe, B.H., Jimpson, G., and Michela, N.J. (1992). Low-income program increases mammography compliance. *Oncology Nursing Forum*, 19(5): p. 822.

Epperson, Z. (1991). The story of a downwinder. In Judith Brady, *1 in 3: Women with cancer confront an epidemic*. San Francisco, CA: Cleis Press, pp. 89-96.

Freire, P. (1990). *Pedagogy of the oppressed*. New York: Continuum.

Garland, J.A., Jones, H.E., and Kolodny, R.L. (1976). A model for stages of development in social work groups. In S. Bernstein, *Explorations in group work*. Boston, MA: Practitioner, pp. 17-71.

Gawler, I. (1987). *You can conquer cancer*. Rochester, NY: Thorsons.

Germain, C.P. (1979). *The cancer unit: An ethnography*. Wakefield, MA: Nursing Resources.

Gilbar, O. (1991). Model for crisis intervention through group therapy for women with breast cancer. *Clinical Social Work Journal*, 19(3): pp. 293-304.

Gilbert, M.C. (1990). Developing a group program in a health care setting. In J.H. Schopler and M.J. Galinsky, *Groups in health care settings*. Binghamton, NY: The Haworth Press, Inc., pp. 27-44.

Goldberg, R.J. and Tull, R.M. (1983). *The psychosocial dimensions of cancer: A practical guide for health care providers*. New York: Free Press.

Hagen, J.L. and Davis, L.V. (1992). Working with women: Building a policy and practice agenda. *Social Work Journal of the National Association of Social Workers*, 37(6): pp. 481-576.

Hardisty, J. and Leopold, E. (1992). Cancer and poverty: Double jeopardy for women. *Sojourner: The women's forum,* 6, December: pp. 14-18. Reprinted by permission.

Haskell, C.M. (1990). *Cancer treatment.* Philadelphia, PA: Harcourt, Brace, Jovanovich.

Hickey, S.J. (1989). Hope as a key element in cancer survivorship. *Journal of Psychosocial Oncology,* 7(4): pp 111-118.

Hubner, M.K. (1989). Cancer and infertility: Longing for life. *Journal of Psychosocial Oncology,* 7(4): pp. 1-19.

Jampolsky, G.G. (1989). Out of darkness into the light: A journey of inner healing. New York: Bantam.

Kendall, J. (Ed.). (1993). Making sense of scents. Citizens for a toxic-free Marin.

Kofron, E.E. (1993). The language of cancer. *Family Therapy Networker,* 17(1): pp. 35-43.

Kosa, J., Antonovsky, A., and Zola, I.K. (Eds.). (1969). *Poverty and health.* London: Oxford Press.

Love, Richard R. (1989). Tamoxifen therapy in primary breast cancer: Biology, efficacy, and side effects. *Journal of Clinical Oncology,* 7(6): pp. 803-815.

Lum, D. (1986). *Social work practice and people of color: A process-stage approach.* Monterey, CA: Brooks/Cole.

McFate, P. (1979). Ethical issues in the treatment of cancer patients. In B.R. Cassileth, *The cancer patient.* Philadelphia, PA: Lea and Febiger, pp. 59-74.

McGinn, K.A. and Haylock, P.J. (1993). *Women's cancers: How to prevent them how to treat them how to beat them.* Alameda, CA: Hunter House.

McGregor, M. (1993). Harvest of a silent spring. *Breast Cancer Action,* August (19): pp. 7-11.

Mellette, S.J. (1989). Rehabilitation issues for cancer survivors—Psychosocial challenges. *Journal of Psychosocial Oncology,* 7(4): pp. 93-103.

Memik, F., Gulten, M., and Nak, S.G. (1992). The etiological role of diet, smoking, and drinking habits of patients with esophageal carcinoma in Turkey. *Journal of Environmental Pathology, Toxicology, and Oncology,* 11(4): pp. 197-200.

Menchaca, M. (1989). Chicano-Mexican cultural assimilation and Anglo-Saxon cultural dominance. *The Hispanic Journal of Behavioral Sciences,* 2(3): pp. 203-231.

Millichap, J.D. (1993). *Environmental poisons in our food.* Chicago, IL: PNB Publishers.

Mor, V., Allen, S.M., Siegel, K., and Houts, P. (1992). Determinants of need and unmet need among cancer patients residing at home. *Health Services Research,* 27(3): pp. 337-360.

Moss, R.W. (1989). *The cancer industry.* New York: Paragon House.

New York Coalition for Alternatives to Pesticides (NYCAP). (1993). *NYCAP News,* 4(1).

Northern, H. (1990). Social work practice with groups in health care. In J.H. Schopler and M.J. Galinsky, *Groups in health care settings.* Binghamton, NY: The Haworth Press, Inc., pp. 7-26.

Null, G., Sternglass, E., and Gould, J. (1993). What physicians should know about the biological effects of ingested fission products. *Townsend Letter for Doctors: An Informal Letter Magazine for Doctors Communicating with Doctors,* August/September: pp. 121-122.

Pelzer, A., Duncan, M.E., Tibau, G., and Mehari, L. (1992). A study of cervical cancer in Ethiopian women. *Cytopathology,* 3(3): pp. 139-148.

Physicians' Desk Reference. (1993). Edition 47. Montvale, NJ: Medical Economics Data.

Reid, P.T. (1993). Poor women in psychological research: Shut up and shut out. *Psychology of Women Quarterly,* 17: pp. 133-150.

Reyes, L. (1991). Study group report: Chemotherapy. *Breast Cancer Action Newsletter,* 1(4), p. 2. Breast Cancer Action, 55 New Montgomery Street, Suite 323, San Francisco, CA 94105 (415) 243-9301.

Samuels, M.D. and Samuels, N. (1988). *Seeing with the mind's eye.* New York: Random House.

Schopler, J.H. and Galinski, M.J. (1990). Introduction: Social group work: Promoting a more holistic approach to health care. In J.H. Schopler and M.J. Galinsky, *Groups in health care settings.* Binghamton, NY: The Haworth Press, Inc., pp. 1-6.

Schopler, J.H. and Galinsky, M.J. (1993). Support groups as open systems: A model for practice and research. *Health and Social Work,* 18(3): pp. 195-207.

Schultz, W.C. (1950). *FIRO: A three-dimensional theory of interpersonal orientations.* New York: Holt, Rinehart and Winston.

Shalinsky, W. (1967). Group composition as an element of social group work practice. Doctoral Dissertation. Study based on W.C. Schultz's theory of FIRO. Cleveland, OH: School of Applied Social Sciences, Case Western Reserve University.

Siegel, B.S. (1989). *Peace, love and healing.* New York: Harper & Row.

Steingraber, S. (1991). We all live downwind. In Judith Brady, *1 in 3: Women with cancer confront an epidemic.* San Francisco, CA: Cleis Press, pp. 36-48.

Stocker, M. (Ed.). (1993). *Confronting cancer, constructing change: New perspectives on women and cancer.* Chicago, IL: Third Side Press.

Stoll, B.A. (1979). *Mind and cancer prognosis.* Chichester, England: John Wiley and Sons.

Sung, J.F., Coates, R.J., Williams, J.E., Liff, J.M., and Greenberg, R.S. (1992). Cancer screening intervention among black women in inercity Atlanta: Design of a study. In *Public Health Reports,* 107(4), July-August: pp. 381-388.

Takaki, R. (Ed.). (1987). *From different shores: Perspectives in race and ethnicity in America.* New York: Oxford University Press.

Tanne, J.H. (1993). Everything you need to know about breast cancer. *New York,* 26(40): pp. 52-61.

Vernon, S.W., Vogel, V.G., Halabi, S., Jackson, G.L., and Lundy, R.O. (1992). Breast cancer screening behaviors and attitudes in three racial/ethnic groups. In *Cancer,* 69(1), January: pp. 165-174.

Wallas, C. (1991). A puzzling plague: What is it about the American way of life that causes breast cancer? *Time,* January (14): pp. 48-54.

Watson, M., Greer, S., and Thomas, C. (Eds.). (1988). *Psychosocial oncology.* London: Pergamon Press.

Weaver, D. (1982). Empowering treatment skills for helping Black families. *The Journal of Contemporary Social Work,* February: pp. 100-105.

Weisman, H. and Worden, J.W. (1975). Psychosocial analysis of cancer death. In *Journal of Death and Dying,* 6(1): pp. 61-74.

Yancik, R. (1989). Assessing the quality of life of cancer patients: Practical issues in study implementation. *Journal of Psychosocial Oncology,* 7(4): pp. 59-65.

Zemore, R. (1989). Some social and emotional consequences of breast cancer and mastectomy: A content analysis of eighty-seven interviews. *Journal of Psychosocial Oncology,* 7(4): pp. 33-41.

Index

Acceptance, 42
ACS. *See* American Cancer Society
ADA. *See* Americans with
        Disabilities Act
Adriamycin (Doxorubicin), 12,29
American Cancer Society (ACS), 68
American Psychiatric Association, 16
Americans with Disabilities Act,
        23-24
Anderson, B.L., 3,5,6,52
Arditte, R., 65,66
Ativan, 32

Bacon, C., 4
BCA. *See* Breast Cancer Action
Bell, D.S., 85
Belle, D., 4,7,52
Benadryl, 32
Berger, R.M., 69,71,75
Berkow, R., 11,69
Bertcher, H., 55
Brady, J., 14,65,68,71,72
Breast cancer, 66-67
    Maria, 27-39
Breast Cancer Action (BCA), 62-63

Cancer
    breast cancer. *See* Breast cancer
    community models
        Breast Cancer Action (BCA),
            62-63
        Charlotte Maxwell
            Complementary Clinic,
            The, 59-60
        Women's Cancer Resource
            Center, The, 60-62

Cancer *(continued)*
    coping with, 49. *See also* Therapy
    detection (early) of, 66
    diagnosis, 20,35
        stage of at, 57
    and discrimination, 14
    and employment, 14,29
    and fear. *See* Fear
    government agencies for, 77-81
    helping women with, 26
    and lifestyle changes, 20
    and low-income women, *ix*,25
        delaying treatment of, 3
        emotional support for, 20-21,26.
            See also Support group;
            Therapy
        needs of, basic, 48
        oppression of, 57
        stigmatization of, 4-5
    prevention, 65-75
    and social work, 65-75
        credo of social workers, 83-84
    stigma of, 22,52
    support group, 16-17
        planning, 51-58
    surviving, 14
    treatment of
        chemotherapy, fear of, 16
        and drugs. *See individual
            listings*
        and friendships during, 14
Cancer Industry, The, 73
Cancer Rehabilitation, 17
*Cancer-Prevention Resource
        Directory,* 73
Case management, 47-49. *See also*
        Therapy
Cassileth, B.R., 52